In the name of Allah, the most

Compassionate, the most Merciful.

Dedicated to

Professor (Hakim) Syed Zillur Rahman Sahib

for your continuing love and support, and for

continuing to shine the light of Unani Tibb.

Acknowledgements

The following people have read and commented on the draft of the book, pointed out mistakes and made suggestions for improvements: Syed Abdul H. Qadri Sahib, Meher Alam Khan Sahib, Sumera Khan. My special thanks to Hussein Ahmed for his tireless help and support without which this book would not have been published. I also thank Ainsley Macadam for her valuable feedback on the 1st edition.

The Golden Key to Discovering Yourself

by

M. Salim Khan

M.D. (M.A.) M.H. D.O.

M.I.R.C.H. F.G.N.I.

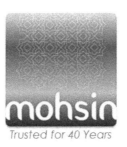

Trusted for 40 Years

Published by Mohsin Health

446 East Park Road, Leicester, LE5 5HH, UK

Website: www.mohsinhealth.co.uk

E-mail: info@mohsinhealth.co.uk

22 Jumada-al-Awwal 1440 AH

28 January 2019 CE

2nd edition published

in January 2019

© M Salim Khan

Published by: Mohsin Health

446 East Park Road, Leicester, LE5 5HH, UK

Website: www.mohsinhealth.co.uk

E-mail: info@mohsinhealth.co.uk

ISBN-13: 978-0-9929456-1-9

مَنْ عَرَفَ نَفْسَهُ فَقَدْ عَرَفَ رَبَّهُ

"man ʿarafa nafsahu faqad ʿarafa Rabbahu"

"Whosoever knows himself knows his Lord."

ΓΝΩΘΙ
ΣΑΥΤΟΝ

"Know Thyself"

Contents

Introduction

From the earliest times in human history, across various cultures and civilisations, uniqueness and individuality of each person has been at the centre of health and wellbeing. This concept, called temperament, is found in all healthcare traditions and has been used and applied universally throughout history. The aim of this book is to provide 'The Golden Key' to help unlock the hidden treasures within each of us as individuals. We will be reconnecting with the lost wisdom and knowledge of humanity, our heritage which stretches over the last five millennia. Understanding our own unique, individual temperament or personality type will facilitate us to tune into the vast treasures of knowledge within the healthcare traditions of Africa, China, India, Europe and Arabia. This reconnection with the sacred knowledge, together with accumulated experience of humanity, brings us towards wholeness and balance. Understanding temperament helps us to make sense of all of the available information and data, which is meaningless without this framework. This helps us to achieve higher health, wellbeing and enlightenment.

M. Salim Khan – 28th January 2019, Leicester, UK

Part One:

The Current Health Crisis

1. The Current Health Crisis

"At the beginning of the last two decades of our century, we find ourselves in a state of profound, world-wide crisis. It is a complex, multi-dimensional crisis whose facets touch every aspect of our lives - our health and our livelihood, the quality of our environment and our social relationships, our economy, technology and politics. It is a crisis of intellectual, moral and spiritual dimensions of a scale and urgency unprecedented in recorded human history. Fritjof Capra in his book *The Turning Point*

Our Crazy Lifestyles – Humanity Stuck in a Rut

We live in a post-modern, post-industrial age in which the Earth is being poisoned and destroyed. Post-modern lifestyle, with all its apparent glitter and conveniences, poisons and depletes our body, mind, spirit and relationships. We are being forced away from our pure, unadulterated nature – Fiṭra. Instead, we are experiencing poor health and increase in numbers of degenerative diseases, leading to:

1. Depleted energy.
2. Poor relationships.
3. Social isolation.
4. Inability to be of service.

5. Poverty and low earning ability.

6. Lack of enjoyment in life.

7. Negative self-image.

8. Dependency on poor public healthcare.

9. Becoming victim of toxic drugs (legal addictions).

10. Spiritual depletion.

Chronic diseases are causing millions of premature deaths yearly, as well as sabotaging quality of life for hundreds of millions more. Public healthcare is in crisis and our cherished and loved healthcare institutions are becoming dysfunctional and breaking down.

Beginning of the Industrial Revolution

Industrial lifestyle and medicine can be traced back to the industrial revolution which began to introduce much of this harm.

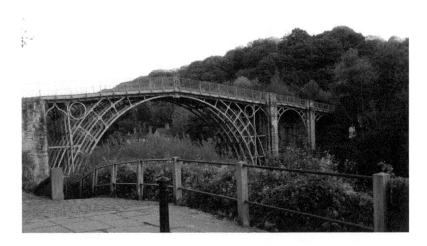

Pictured above is a symbol of the industrial revolution, the Iron Bridge, which crosses the River Severn in Shropshire, England. Opened in 1781, it was the first major bridge in the world to be made of cast iron, and was greatly celebrated after construction.

Poisonous Fruits of the Industrial Revolution

One of the consequences of the industrial revolution is the pollution and poisoning of the natural environment.

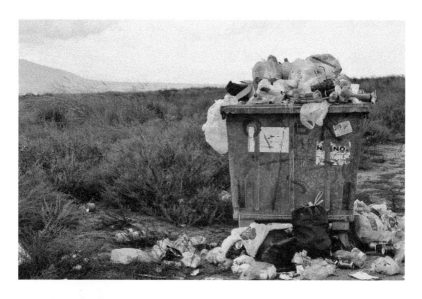

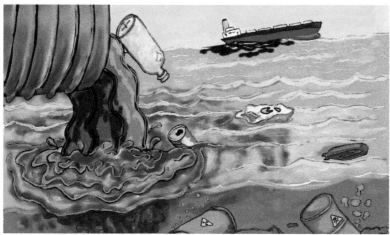

Post-Industrial Times

In the post-industrial world, industrial values have accelerated more and more with the latest technologies and discoveries.

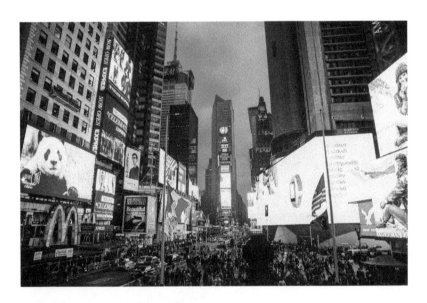

Post-Industrial Junk Food

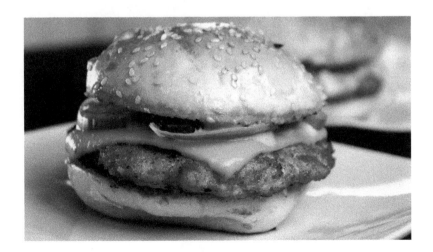

Post-Modern, Post-Industrial Lifestyle

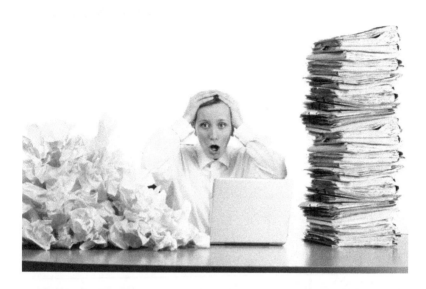

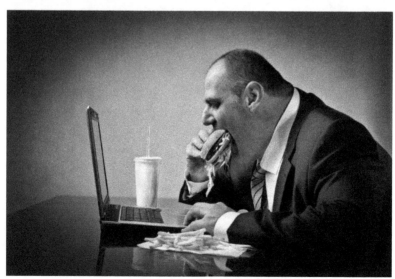

Enslavement to Modern Diseases

The term 'Western diseases' encompasses a large group of disease. These wide variety of human ailments are also known as non-communicable diseases, or NCDs. By definition, NCDs are also known as chronic diseases or lifestyle diseases, not passed on from person to person. They are of long duration and generally have a slow progression.

The four main categories of NCDs are:

1. Cardiovascular
2. Cancers
3. Chronic respiratory diseases
4. Diabetes

These four main groups of diseases account for around 80% of all deaths caused by NCDs. NCDs are projected to exceed the combined deaths caused by communicable and nutritional diseases, as well as maternal and perinatal deaths. NCDs are projected to be the most common cause of death in the world by 2030.

Cardiovascular diseases account for the highest percentage of deaths caused by NCDs (17.3 million people annually, worldwide), followed by cancer (7.6 million), respiratory diseases (4.2 million), and diabetes (1.3 million).

There is growing awareness and reliable research evidence, across various disciplines, which shows that degradation in the environment, lifestyle and diet is leading to chronic diseases and untold human suffering.

These changes have accelerated since the industrial revolution. As they have become so rapid and widespread, these changes have placed human beings and the natural environment into serious disturbance and chaos. There is now a manifest discordance between natural human needs and the environment.

The discordance is particularly manifest in contemporary lifestyles, diet and nutrition. The last 200 years of systematic cross-cultural research have identified seven main changes in the dietary and nutritional field. These are all deviations from traditional dietary patterns.

Of the 56.9 million deaths worldwide in 2016, more than half (54%) were due to the top 10 causes. Heart disease and stroke are the world's biggest killers, accounting for a combined 15.2 million deaths in 2016.

Chronic obstructive pulmonary disease claimed 3.0 million lives in 2016, while lung cancer (along with trachea and bronchus cancers) caused 1.7 million deaths. Diabetes killed 1.6 million people in 2016, up from less than 1 million in 2000.

Top 10 global causes of deaths, 2016

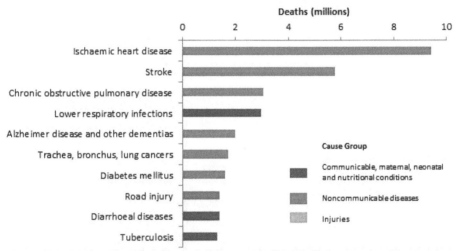

Source: Global Health Estimates 2016: Deaths by Cause, Age, Sex, by Country and by Region, 2000-2016. Geneva, World Health Organization; 2018.

The Cure is Worse than the Disease

An example of a so-called 'magic bullet' and its damaging consequences is thalidomide. This pharmaceutical drug was marketed as a mild sleeping pill safe even for pregnant women, however it caused thousands of babies worldwide to be born with malformed limbs. [1]

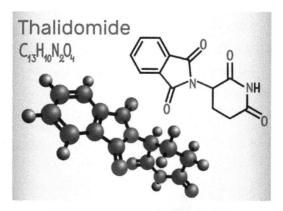

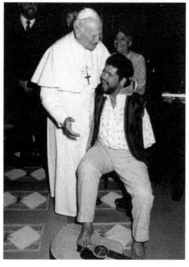

The Crisis of Modern Industrial Medicine

Since the renaissance in European societies, the fundamental conceptions of creation of life and the human being have developed on mechanistic and materialistic lines to the exclusion of any higher values. This materialistic and mechanistic view of the world professes that 'God is dead' for all significant intents and purposes.

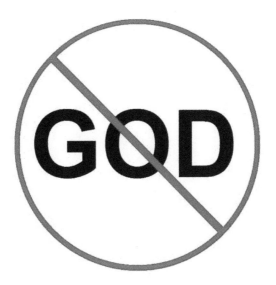

This view of the world has created fundamental problems for human beings, including in the area of health and wellbeing. This reductionist approach produces the erroneous belief that disease is the result of a single causative factor – for example 'germs'. It is based on this belief that industrial medicine is in search of a 'magic bullet' to cure diseases.

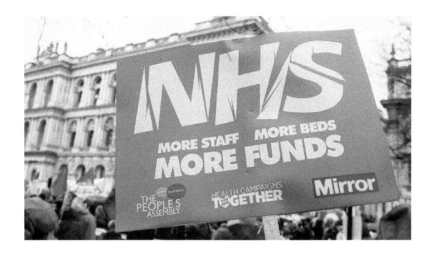

Modern industrial medicine, after dazzling the world for 200 years, is now suffering with a crisis of confidence. This crisis is particularly widespread in the UK, Europe and USA. Some of the reasons are:

1. Dehumanisation and commoditisation of patients and healthcare professionals.
2. Industrial medicine is expensive, sapping the financial resources of nations.
3. Its participation in helping to sustain the epidemic of chronic lifestyle diseases.
4. The phenomenal, unacceptable increase in iatrogenic diseases.
5. Re-emergence of life-threatening infections due to abuse of antibiotics.

Healthcare Breaking Down

As mentioned previously, our cherished and loved healthcare institutions are crumbling, such as the NHS (National Health Service) in the United Kingdom.

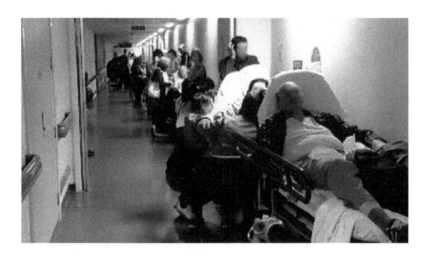

The picture above, posted online, shows a hospital in Staffordshire, UK, where emergency facilities were overwhelmed. A huge queue of patients on trolleys stretched into the distance at this hospital's A&E (accident and emergency) department.

Crisis in Public Healthcare – Britain as an Example

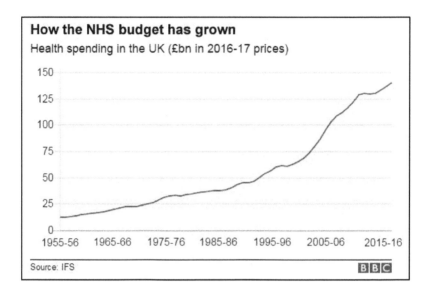

How the NHS budget has grown

Health spending in the UK (£bn in 2016-17 prices)

Source: IFS

BBC

We spend more on the NHS than ever before. Last year £140bn was spent on health across the UK - more than 10 times the figure that was spent 60 years ago (after taking into account inflation). [2]

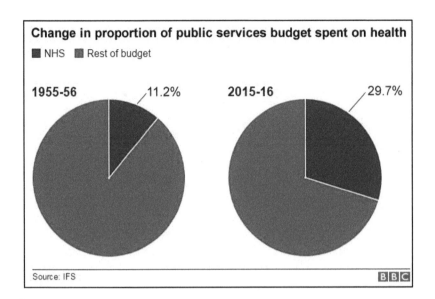

Source: IFS

A bigger proportion of public spending goes on health. Governments over the years have had to invest more and more of the public purse into it. Today 30p out of every £1 spent on services goes on health.

Even during the years of deep austerity, extra money has been found for the health service. Yet it seems no matter how much is invested, it's still not enough. The NHS is creaking at the seams. [3]

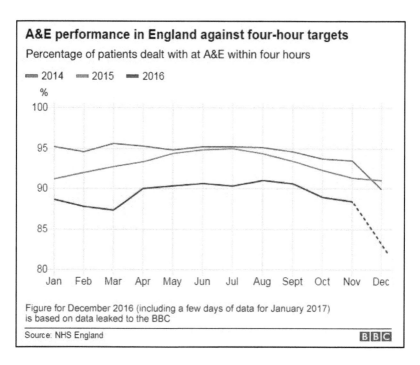

A&E performance in England against four-hour targets

Percentage of patients dealt with at A&E within four hours

2014   2015   2016

Figure for December 2016 (including a few days of data for January 2017) is based on data leaked to the BBC

Source: NHS England   BBC

Key A&E (accident and emergency) targets are being missed. The barometer of this is the four-hour A&E target. This is a sign of whether the system is under stress - both in the community and in the hospital. Demand for A&E is rising. The numbers visiting A&E have risen by a third in 12 years. Two-thirds of hospitals beds are occupied by people with chronic conditions. [4]

Doctors Burning Out

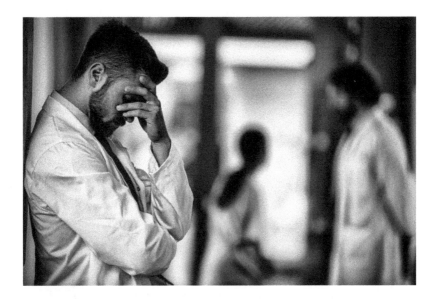

Research by the University of Exeter Medical School has found GPs are "fed up" with "unlimited demands" on them. Doctors spoke of concerns about the risk of litigation and problems with their own health due to work pressures.

Dr Richard Vautrey, chair of the British Medical Association GPs committee, said: "This is a crisis which we've been pointing out for a number of years." He said the BMA was regularly contacted by GPs who are concerned about workload pressures. "They feel they're not able to provide safe patient care."

The number of full-time equivalent GPs fell by 1,193 in the year up to October 2017, compared to a drop of 97 the year before, according to NHS Digital. In October 2017, there were 33,302 full-time equivalent GPs in England, compared to 34,495 the year before.

Dr Linda Thomas quit general practice in Bristol to set up an eco-fashion company. She said: "At the worst stages I would come back from a long surgery and I would be physically shaking because the pressure of trying to meet the needs of all the people, the time pressure, the system pressure, just became so hard... I'm a mum as well. I need to be a whole human being. I can't just be a medic and then nothing." [5]

The Need for an Alternative

Moving Away from Poisonous and Chaotic Lifestyles to Sustainable Alternatives

"Contemporary Western men and women, in quest of the sacred and the rediscovery of pontifical man, seek techniques of meditation which overcome the excessive cerebral activity which characterises modern mental activity, allowing the agitated mind to simply be. The quest may include yoga, oriental forms of medicine, natural food and medicine and the like. In reality the quest is for the heart which, in the spiritual person, who is aware of his vocation as man, 'penetrates' into both the head and the body, integrating them into the centre, bestowing a contemplative perfume to mental activity and intellectual and spiritual presence to the body, which is reflected in its gestures and motion." Fritjof Capra

Getting Out of the Rut

The public are seeking alternative healthcare solutions worldwide. Consequently, the last few decades have seen a resurgence of various forms of natural medicine and healing. Some of these are long established traditions such as Ayurveda, Unani Tibb, and traditional Chinese medicine, which go back thousands of years. Others, such as osteopathy and reflexology, are relatively new. These diverse forms of natural medicine and healing are lumped together by dominant establishments under the label of 'complementary and alternative medicine', or CAM. The dominant medical establishment including pharmaceutical complex continues to attack CAM, claiming:

1. It is unscientific
2. It is ineffective
3. It is unsafe and dangerous
4. Practitioners of CAM are 'quacks' and charlatans
5. They are money making schemes and scams

However, the growth of CAM and of wisdom-based traditions of healthcare and medicine continues, particularly noticeable within industrial and post-industrial societies of Europe and USA. One of the distinctive features of natural and traditional medicines is that they are an integral part of man's philosophy, his consciousness and his relationships with other beings and the cosmos. The emphasis of oneness and unity enable connectedness and not disintegration, which is often the hallmark of drug and surgery-based methods. The consequence of a wholistic perspective is human development and inter-connectedness.

The Unity of the Person

Unani Tibb has an integrated approach towards health and disease. This means a wholistic view and seeing the whole of life and the human being as an integrated totality – Waḥda. In practice, this means any disease or imbalance disturbs the whole person. In dealing with health and wellbeing, the unity of the person must be kept in mind.

Dimensions of the Human Being

There is a hierarchy of gradation within each human being. The four primary levels are:

- Spiritual
- Emotional
- Mental
- Physical

Turning Humans into Machines

As a reaction to the exploitation and abuse by religious authorities, specifically in Europe, there was a revolt against God and religion per se. This revolt and rebellion against humanity's accumulated wisdom and knowledge has lead to 'modern science' becoming a new, Godless ideology that tramples over all earlier human achievements in the name of 'progress' and scientism. This has led to dehumanisation of the individual, treating humans as unconscious, purposeless and expendable machines.

Today, most (if not all) research is done from mechanical perspectives. There is a plethora of facts, figures and information about everything under the Sun. In the area of health and disease, there is conflicting information from various agencies and experts leading to confusion and increasing burden of disease. Until we replace this industrial model with a person-centred and individualised approach, things are likely to deteriorate even further.

Rediscovering the Uniqueness of Each Individual

This book will explore the common theme of temperaments found in major wisdom-based traditions of healthcare and medicine. This will help us to rediscover each of our own unique individuality. Particularly, in this book, we will be looking at temperament as seen from within Unani Tibb. Our focus will be how we can improve and transform our health using the rich reservoirs of experience, wisdom and knowledge found in this particular tradition.

"For the first time we have to face the real threat of extinction of the human race and all life on this planet." Fritjof Capra in his book *The Turning Point*

Part Two:

Historical Background

2. Traditional Chinese Understanding of Temperament

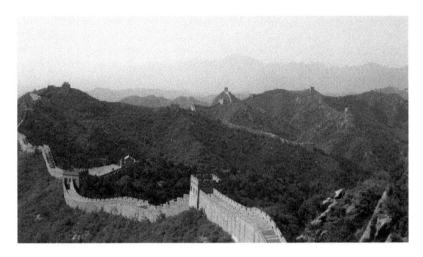

The concept of Yin-Yang is probably the single most important and distinctive theory of Chinese medicine. It could be said that all Chinese medical physiology, pathology and treatment can, eventually, be reduced to Yin-Yang. [6] The concept of Yin-Yang is extremely simple, yet very profound. One can seemingly understand it on a rational level and yet, continually find new expressions of it in clinical practice and, indeed, in life.

Application of Yin and Yang to Medicine

It could be said that the whole of Chinese medicine, its physiology, pathology, diagnosis and treatment, can all be reduced to the basic and fundamental theory of Yin and Yang.

Every physiological process and every symptom or sign can be analysed in the light of the Yin and Yang theory. Ultimately, every treatment modality is aimed at one of these four strategies:

1. To tonify Yang.
2. To tonify Yin.
3. To eliminate excess Yang.
4. To eliminate excess Yin.

Understanding the application of the theory of Yin-Yang to medicine is therefore of supreme importance in practice. One can say that there is no Chinese medicine without Yin-Yang.

"Yin and Yang, the two principles in nature and the four seasons are the beginning and the end of everything, and they are also the cause of life and death. Those who disobey the laws of the universe will give rise to calamities and visitations, while those who follow the laws of the universe remain free from dangerous illness." The Yellow Emperor's Classic of Internal Medicine

Yin-Yang and Body Structure

Every part of the human body has a predominantly Yin or Yang character, and this is important in clinical practice. It must be emphasised, however, that this character is only relative. For example, the chest area is Yang in relation to the abdomen (because it is higher) but Yin in relation to the head.

As a general rule, the following are the characters of various body structures:

Yang	Yin
Superior	Inferior
Exterior	Interior
Posterior (Lateral Surface)	Anterior (Medial Surface)
Back	Front
Function	Structure

More specifically, the Yin-Yang characters of the body structures, organs and energies are:

Yang	Yin
Back	Front (Chest and Abdomen)
Head	Body
Exterior (Skin and Muscles)	Interior (Internal Organs)
Above The Waist	Below The Waist
Posterior (Lateral Surface of Limbs)	Interior (Medial Surface of Limbs)
Yang Organs	Yin Organs
Function of Organs	Structure of Organs
Qi	Blood-Body Fluids
Defensive Qi	Nutritive Qi

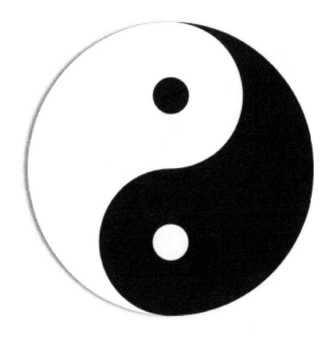

(Fig. 1) Yin and Yang Symbol

Application of Key Principles of Yin-Yang to Medicine

We can look at a few core principles to show the following relationships:

- Opposition of Yin-Yang
- The Inter-Transformation of Yin-Yang [7]

Opposition of Yin-Yang

The opposition of Yin-Yang is reflected in medicine in the opposing Yin-Yang structures of the human body, the opposing Yin-Yang character of the organs and most of all, in the opposing symptomatology of Yin and Yang. No matter how complicated, all symptoms and signs in Chinese medicine can be reduced to their elemental, basic character of Yin or Yang. In order to interpret the character of the clinical manifestations in terms of Yin-Yang, we can refer to certain basic qualities which will guide us in clinical practice, shown in the table on the next page.

Yang	Yin
Fire	Water
Hot	Cold
Restless	Quiet
Dry	Wet
Hard	Soft
Excitement	Inhibition
Rapidity	Slowness
Non-substantial	Substantial
Transformation, change	Conservation, storage, sustainment

(Fig. 2) Yin-Yang Qualities

Some of the Yin-Yang qualities are explained further below.

Fire-Water

This is one of the fundamental dualities of Yin-Yang in Chinese medicine. Although these terms derive from the Five Element Theory, there is an interaction between that and the theory of Yin-Yang

The balance between fire and water in the body is crucial. Fire is essential to all physiological processes. It represents the flame that keeps alive and stokes all metabolic processes.

Fire assists the heart in its function of housing the mind. It provides the warmth necessary for the spleen to transform and transport. It stimulates the small intestine's function of separation, and provides the heat necessary to the bladder and lower burner to transform and excrete fluids.

If the physiological fire declines, the mind will suffer with depression, and the spleen cannot transform and transport. The small intestine cannot separate the fluids and there will be oedema.

This physiological fire is called 'the fire of the gate of vitality' – and derives from the kidneys.

Water has the function of moistening and cooling during all the body's physiological functions, in order to balance the warming action of the physiological fire. The origin of water is also from the kidneys.

Thus, the balance between fire and water is fundamental to all physiological processes of the body. Fire and water balance and keep check of each other in every single physiological process.

When fire gets out of hand and becomes excessive, it has a tendency to flow upwards, hence the manifestations will show on the top part of the body and head, with headaches, red eyes, red face or thirst. When water becomes excessive, it has a tendency to flow downwards causing oedema of the legs, excessive urination or incontinence.

Hot-Cold

Excess of Yang is manifested with heat and excess of Yin is manifested with cold. For example, a person with excess of Yang will feel hot, and one with excess of Yin will tend to feel cold.

The hot and cold character can also be observed in certain signs themselves. For example, a large single boil that is red and hot to the touch indicates heat. A lower back area very cold to the touch indicates cold in the kidneys.

Dry-Wet

Any symptom or sign of dryness such as dry eyes, dry throat, dry skin or dry stools, indicates excess of Yang (or deficiency of Yin). Any symptom or sign of excess wetness such as watery eyes, runny nose, damp pimples on the skin or loose stools, indicates excess of Yin (or deficiency of Yang).

Hard-Soft

Any lumps, swellings or masses that are hard are usually due to excess of Yang, whereas if they are soft they are due to excess of Yin.

The Inter-Transformation of Yin-Yang

Although they are opposite, Yin and Yang can change into one another. This transformation does not take place at random, but is determined by the stage of development and by internal conditions.

First of all, the change takes place when conditions are ripe at a certain point in time. Day cannot turn into night at any time, but only when it has reached its point of exhaustion.

The second condition of change is determined by the internal qualities of any given thing or phenomenon. Wood can turn into coal, but a stone cannot. The process of transformation of Yin and Yang into each other can be observed in many natural phenomena, such as in the alternation of day and night, the seasons and climate.

The principle of inter-transformation of Yin-Yang has many applications in clinical practice. An understanding of this transformation is important for the prevention of disease. If we are aware of how a thing can turn into its opposite, then we can prevent this and achieve a balance which is the essence of Chinese medicine.

For example, excessive work (Yang) without rest induces extreme deficiency (Yin) of the body's energies. Excessive jogging (Yang) induces a very slow (Yin) pulse. Excessive consumption of alcohol creates a pleasant euphoria (Yang) which is quickly followed by a hang-over (Yin). Excessive worrying (Yang) depletes (Yin) the energy of the body.

Thus, balance in our life, in diet, exercise, work, emotional life and sexual life, is the essence of prevention in Chinese medicine and an understanding of how Yang can turn into Yin and vice versa can help us to avoid the rapid swings from one to the other which are detrimental to our physical and emotional life.

Of course, nothing would be more difficult to achieve in our modern societies, which seem to be geared to producing the maximum swing from one extreme to the other. [8]

"In ancient times those people who understood the Tao (self discipline) patterned themselves upon the Yin and the Yang (two principles in nature) and they lived in harmony. There was temperance in eating and drinking. Their hours of rising and retiring were regular and not disorderly and wild." The Nei Ching

3. Ayurvedic Understanding of Temperament

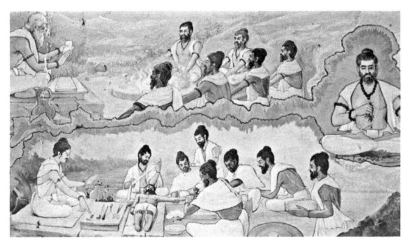

Ayurveda, a wholistic system of medicine indigenous to India is estimated to have been practised since 2500 BCE. [9] According to Ayurveda, there are five Elements: Ether, Air, Fire, Water and Earth. These manifest as three basic principles, known as Tridosha (or three Doshas). According to Ayurveda, the basic Prakruti – nature of an individual, is largely determined at conception. The following pages give a description of the three primary types of temperament according to Ayurveda. [10] [11]

All Ayurvedic literature is based on the Samkhya philosophy of creation. According to this paradigm, the universe evolved of Avyakta – the unmanifested. Purusha – primordial consciousness is beyond attributes and takes no active part in the manifestation of the universe.

Prakruti – literally meaning nature, creates all forms in the universe. It is the primordial energy which contains the three Gunas – qualities. Together known as Trigunas, they are:

- Sativa – knowledge, happiness, white
- Rajas – activity, pain, red
- Tamas – resistance, intertia, confusion, dark

One of the basic tenets of Ayurveda is that the human being is a microcosm of the very world he inhabits. This implies that whatever the human being is made up of, the world too is made up of those same constituents, elements or forces, but of different combinations and degrees.

Mahabutas – the five elements are: Akasa – Ether; Vayu – Air; Tejas – Fire; Ap – Water; Prithvi – Space/Earth.

Each person's Prakruti – individual nature or constitution is unique. In Ayurvedic practice, it is the Dosha which is the individual's temperament.

Vata Temperament

Physical

People of Vata temperament are generally physically underdeveloped. Their chests are flat and their veins and muscle tendons are visible.

Vata complexion is brown; the skin is cold, rough, dry and cracked. There usually are a few moles present, which tend to be dark.

Vata people are generally either too tall or too short, with thin frames which reveal prominent joints and bone-ends because of poor muscle development.

The hair is curly and scanty, the eye lashes are thin and the eyes lustreless. The eyes may be sunken, small, dry, active and the conjunctiva is dry and muddy.

The nails are rough and brittle. The shape of the nose is bent and turned up.

Psychological

Psychologically they are characterised by short memory but quick mental understanding. They will understand something immediately, but will soon forget it.

They have little will power, tend toward mental instability and possess little tolerance, confidence or boldness. Their reasoning power is weak and these people are nervous, fearful and afflicted by much anxiety.

Physiological

Physiologically, the appetite and digestion are variable. Vata people crave sweet, sour and salty tastes and like hot drinks. The production of urine is scanty and the faeces are dry, hard and small in quantity.

They have a tendency to perspire less than other temperamental types. Their sleep may be disturbed and they will sleep less than the other types. Their hands and feet are often cold. These people are creative, active, alert and restless.

They talk fast and walk fast but they are easily fatigued. Each temperamental type also exhibits certain patterns in interactions with the external environment. Vata people tend to earn money quickly and also spend it quickly. Thus, they tend to remain poor.

Pitta Temperament

Physical

Physically these people are of medium height, are slender and body frame may be delicate. Their chests are not as flat as those of Vata people and they show a medium prominence of veins and muscle tendons. They have many moles or freckles which are bluish or brownish-red. The bones are not as prominent as in the Vata individual. Muscle development is moderate.

Complexion

Pitta complexion may be coppery, yellowish, reddish or fair. The skin is soft, warm and less wrinkled than Vata skin. The hair is thin, silky, red or brownish and there is a tendency toward premature greying of the hair and hair loss. The eyes may be grey, green or copper brown and sharp; the eyeballs will be of medium prominence. The conjunctiva is moist and copper coloured. The nails are soft. The shape of the nose is sharp and the tip tends to be reddish.

Psychological

Psychologically, Pitta people have a good power of comprehension; they are very intelligent and sharp and tend to be good orators. They have emotional tendencies toward hate, anger and jealousy.

Physiological

Physiologically, these people have a strong metabolism, good digestion and resulting strong appetites. The person of Pitta temperament usually takes large quantities of food and liquid. Pitta types have a natural craving for sweet, bitter and astringent tastes and enjoy cold drinks. Their sleep is of medium duration but uninterrupted. They produce a large volume of urine and the faeces are yellowish, liquid, soft and plentiful. There is a tendency toward excessive perspiring. The body temperature may run slightly high and hands and feet will tend to be warm. Pitta people do not tolerate sunlight, heat or hard work well. They are ambitious people who generally like to be leaders. Pitta people appreciate material prosperity and they tend to be moderately well-off financially. They enjoy exhibiting their wealth and luxurious possessions.

Kapha Temperament

Physical

People of Kapha temperament have well-developed bodies. There is however, a strong tendency for these individuals to carry excess weight. Their chests are expanded and broad. The veins and tendons of Kapha people are not obvious because of their thick skin and their muscle development is good. The bones are not prominent.

Complexion

Kapha complexions are fair and bright. The skin is soft, lustrous and oily; it is also cold and pale. The hair is thick, dark, soft and wavy. The eyes are dense and black or blue; the white of the eye is generally very white, large and attractive. The conjunctiva does not tend to redness.

Physiological

Physiologically, they tend to be tolerant, calm, forgiving and loving; however, they also exhibit traits of greed, attachment, envy and possessiveness. Their comprehension is slow but definite. Once they understand something, that knowledge is retained.

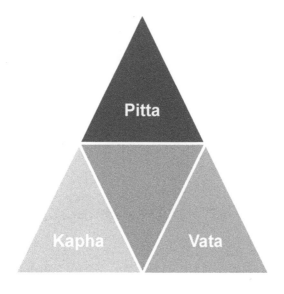

(Fig. 3) The Ayurvedic
Temperaments

4. European Understanding of Temperament

Roots of European Medicine

Ancient Egyptian medicine was the source of a large proportion of European medicine, specifically Greek medicine. Contrary to widespread opinion, ancient Egyptian medicine was of high standard. [12] For example, the Ancient Egyptians had a well-developed four-humour theory in practice when the Greeks had only three. It was Thales of Miletus (640 BCE – 546 BCE) who studied medicine in Egypt and added the fourth humour, Black Bile to the Greek medical system to bring it into line with the Egyptian. [13]

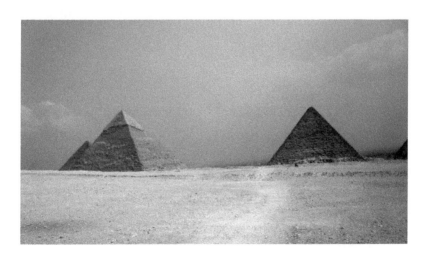

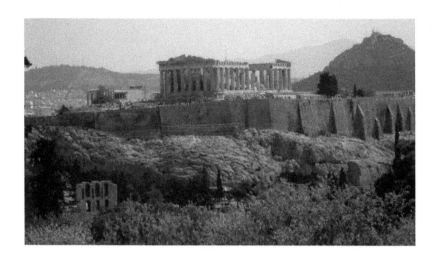

Hippocrates designated two fundamental physical types. He called them the *phthisic habitus* and the *apoplectic habitus*.

The phthisic had a long, thin body, dominated by the vertical dimension. The apoplectic was short, thick individual and strong in the horizontal dimension. Hippocrates thought that the phthisic physique was particularly susceptible to tuberculosis (phthitis).

He knew that the thick, solid individual carried a predisposition for diseases of the vascular system leading to apoplexy. This dichotomy is the prototype for the well-known modern conception of asthenic and pyknic types as described by Kretschmer.

Humoural Understanding

The basis of traditional medicine in the West was the theory of humours which had its roots in Eastern medicine. [14] [15]

The doctrine of the temperaments [16] and their corresponding humours is the oldest theory in European thought. [17] Growing out of the four-part cosmology of Empedocles it has had an almost unbroken history. With relatively few changes it has endured from the dawn of European history down until the industrial revolution. Its original logic rested upon the belief that the human being is a micro-cosmic reflection of nature. They should therefore, in their own being, express all the properties of the cosmos.

Cosmic Element	Qualities	Corresponding Humour	Corresponding Temperament
Fire	Hot and Dry	Yellow Bile	Choleric
Air	Warm and Moist	Blood	Sanguine
Water	Cold and Moist	Phlegm	Phlegmatic
Earth	Cold and Dry	Black Bile	Melancholic

(Fig. 4) Properties of the Four Elements, Corresponding Humours and Temperaments

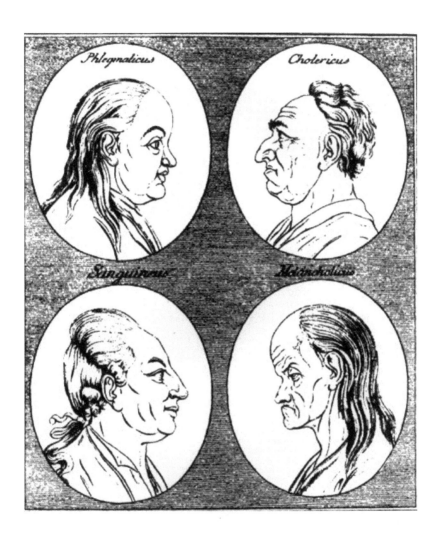

(Fig. 5) The Four Temperaments Illustrated

The classical doctrine ascribed peculiarities of temperament to the 'humours' of the body. Later variations of the theory took form of subdividing or renaming the temperaments, and of modernising the conception of humours. This doctrine profoundly influenced medicine in European societies, especially down to the time of Harvey's re-discovery of blood circulation.

Industrial and Post-Industrial Perspectives

In practice, the concept of temperaments has now been discarded by modern medicine. Instead, there have been numerous attempts by the scientific establishment to classify human beings within the last two hundred years which have resulted in various perspectives, almost all of them inadequate to explain the individuality of each person.

In 1828, Rostan published a famous treatise describing three essentially different types of physical temperament. These became known as the *type digestif*, *type musculaire* and *type cerebral*. The generation which followed felt the impact of a new scientific spirit. Darwin, Huxley, Herbert Spencer and their followers had prepared the ground and the idea of applying a statistical method to the problems of human life.

Classification, measurement and correlation were becoming the order of the day.

About 1885, Di Giovanni founded his school of clinical anthropology at Padua, and his pupil Viola went on to differentiate three morphological types which he called the;

- microsplanchnic;
- normosplanchnic, and;
- macrosplanchnic types.

The names are descriptive. The microsplanchnics are persons with small trunks and relatively long limbs, while the macrosplanchnics have large, heavy bodies and relatively short limbs.

As Viola himself pointed out, the microsplanchnic is the old phthisic habitus, and the macrosplanchnic is the apoplectic habitus. Viola's normosplanchnic is merely an intermediate variation. Hence the important differentiation which Rostan had made between the digestive and muscular types was, for the time being, lost.

Kretschmer's Constitutional Types

Asthenic or Leptosomic Type

Thin, slender, tall and gangly; narrow shoulders; long, narrow, flat ribcage; long, narrow head.

Athletic Type

Broad shoulders; sturdy, high head; impressive ribcage; taut belly; shape of the trunk tapers at the bottom; artificially pronounced muscle definition; big boned.

Pyknic Type

Thick-set, medium build; soft, broad face on short neck sitting between the shoulders; impressive paunch; deep, domed ribcage.

Dysplastic Type

Endocrine dysharmonious or poorly developed without endocrine diseases necessarily being detected. [18]

Aschner's Constitutional Types

The Lymphatic Constitution

This constitution [19] has blue eyes and fair skin. It is equivalent to the sycotic described by Hahneman and the hydrogenoid according to Grauvogel. Blue-eyed people have a constitutional sensitivity of the skin, mucous membranes and nervous system.

Blonde haired people with light coloured eyes have a disposition to lymphatism. Dark haired women with light coloured eyes and excessive hair growth have a tendency to dysmenorrhoea.

The Haematogenic Constitution

Brown eyes, dark skin, brown or black hair. This constitution is equivalent to the billiary or the angiotic according to Mattei or the oxygenoid described by Grauvogel.

The Mixed Constitution

Grey-greenish-brown eyes, light impure skin with pigmented spots, dark hair. This constitution is equivalent to the psora, described by Hahneman or the carbonitrogenic according to Grauvogel. This constitution is generally described dyscratic (unsuitable mixing of body fluids), and since antiquity has been associated with chronic, degenerative diseases, tumours, etc. [20]

Part Three:

Discovering Yourself with

the Four Temperaments

"Understand, for thou art a copy of existence for God, so that nothing of existence is lacking in thee. The throne and the pedestal, are they not in thee? The higher world and the lower world? The cosmos is but a human being on a big scale, and thou, thou art cosmos in miniature." Ibn-al-Banna

"God could have made us all sanguinous, we would have lots of fun, but accomplish little,

He could have made us all melancholics, we would have been organised and chartered, but not very cheerful,

He could have made us all choleric (bilious), we would have been set to lead, but impatient that no one would follow!

He could have made us all phlegmatics, we would have a perfect world, but not much enthusiasm for life,

We need each temperament for the total function of the body, each part should do its work to unify this action and produce harmonious results."

Florence Littauer

5. Unani Tibb: Whole-Person Healthcare & Medicine

In the traditional civilisations of China, India and the Middle East, we find some of the oldest and most time-tested traditions of healthcare and medicine. In Egypt, textbooks on medicine were written by the year 3000 BCE. In India, traditional Indian medicine, known as Ayurveda, was practiced and taught at university level in 700 BCE. In China, Chinese medicine was well established by 700 BCE throughout China, with its roots going back at least to 3000 BCE. A distinctive feature of these various traditions of Eastern medicine is that they are an integral part of man's philosophy, his consciousness and his relationships with other beings and the cosmos. The results are a rich harvest of perspectives and modalities that are unsurpassed both in their profundity and sophistication, as well as being practical, economical and ecologically sustainable.

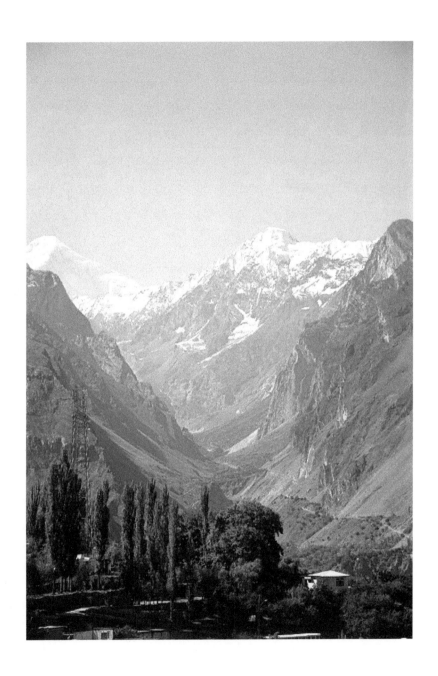

Historical Context

Unani Tibb is a tradition of health, which was synthesised in the crucible of the Middle East, and integrated elements from Egypt, India, China and classical Greece. Unani Tibb is an Arabic name, which in different places has been referred to as Arabic, Greco-Arab, Hikmah, Islamic, and Sufi medicine. Some of the most illustrious names, such as Razi of Persia, Ibn Baytar of Andalusia, Maimonides of Egypt and Ibn Sīnā were practitioners and teachers of Unani Tibb. Today, Unani Tibb continues to provide healthcare for millions of people in India, Pakistan, Afghanistan, Bangladesh, Malaysia and various parts of the Middle East.

Wholeness and Balance

Unani Tibb is a body of knowledge and practice for the purpose of maintaining existing health, and restoring it when lost. Health is a purposeful condition of dynamic balance, in which all the functions are carried out in a correct and whole manner. The concept of wholeness and balance permeates the philosophy, principles and practices of Unani Tibb. In historical times, the condition of wholeness and balance was the norm for most human beings. However, as people and societies moved away from natural patterns, disharmony and diseases increased.

"One of the distinctive features of natural medicines is that they are an integral part of man's philosophy, his consciousness and his relationships with other beings and the cosmos." Fritjof Capra

The wholistic and integrative perspective of Unani Tibb can enable synthesis and development of the individual in the context of the family and the community. The emphasis of oneness and unity enable connectedness and not disintegration, which is often the hallmark of drug and surgery-based methods. The consequence of a wholistic perspective is development and inter-connectedness. In the 21st century the theme of interconnectedness and interdependence will be of psychological and practical significance.

The clarity within the Unani Tibb tradition regards the genesis, nature and purpose of a human being, and provides a vision that is above time and space. It recognises the transcendental aspect of human beings and acknowledges the spiritual nature of each person, which can enable and galvanise individuals towards transformation and unification, an essential need of the 21st Century.

This potential towards transformation and unification constitutes the excellence and zenith of Unani Tibb, a balanced, whole-person medicine. [21]

Theory of Unani Tibb

There are four parts to the theory of Unani Tibb:

1. Umūr-e-Ṭabī'iyya – the 7 aspects of the human constitution – establishes the standards of the human body, from which disease states are deduced by the deviation from these norms.

2. Asbāb-e-Sittah-Ḍharūriyya – literally 'the six essential causative factors', or the theory of causes – which identifies and explains the reasons for deviations from the norms so that they may be corrected.

3. 'Ilm-ul-Amrāz – the theory of signs – which presents the main diagnostic features for identifying the specific deviation that is causing the imbalance and disease.

4. Mu'allijāt – therapeutics – the range and diversity of options for treatment of specific conditions.

Definitions

Definition of Health

Ṣiḥḥah – health is a dynamic condition of I'tidāl – balance in which all the Af'āl – functions are carried out in a Ṣaḥiḥa – correct and Salīma – whole manner.

Definition of Disease

Maraḍ – disease is an abnormal state that primarily disturbs normal functions.

Definition of Medicine

Unani Tibb – whole-person healthcare and medicine – is the body of knowledge and practices that deals with the state of Insān – human beings – in health and disease. Its primary purpose is to maintain health and wellbeing, and endeavour to restore it when lost.

Umūr-e-Ṭabīʿiyya – The 7 Aspects of the Human Constitution

The following are the seven natural dimensions of the human being:

1. Arkān – Elements
2. **Mizāj – Temperament**
3. Akhlāṭ – Humours
4. Aʿḍā – Organs
5. Arwāḥ – Spirits
6. Quwā – Faculties
7. Afʿāl – Functions

The focus of this book is to look at **Mizāj – temperament** in some detail, and how to transform your health and wellbeing. Temperament is the **Golden Key** to discovering and understanding your unique individuality.

6. Unani Tibb Understanding of Mizāj – Temperament

Mizāj – temperament is a dynamic quality that results from mutual actions and interactions of the four primary qualities inherent within the Elements. [22] [23] Temperament as defined above is a unique combination of the physical, emotional, intellectual and spiritual aspects of an individual. It is a dynamic state unique to each individual. Every being is endowed with the most suitable temperament for the purpose and conditions of its creation. Human beings possess the most suitable temperaments for the conditions of life.

Temperament is the inherent predisposition to respond and react along qualitatively predetermined characteristic patterns. Temperamental differences can be observed in the differences of response patterns to identical situations. Each individual responds and reacts according to innate psychological and physiological patterns, many of which they share in common with others, however when combined this set of patterns contributes to the person's unique individuality.

Qualities and Elements

Arkān – the primary Elements – are the simple constituents of minerals, plants and animals. [24] The various orders of creation depend upon intermixtures of the Elements. Throughout the classical civilizations of China, the Middle East, India and Greece, the concept of the Elements has been used to explain and understand nature's most complex processes, including health and disease. Unani Tibb, as a living and dynamic tradition of medicine and healthcare, shares with classical societies the idea of the Elements. However, owing to its own unique historical and social contexts it has its own particular emphasis, which will be the focus of this discussion.

The manifestation of existence by being is a result of polarization of materia prima into Quwā – energy. From the Unani Tibb perspective, the highest levels of organisation of the cosmos are concerned with complex energies. This understanding of the universe also extends to other organisms including human beings. Creating a spectrum for measuring the qualities of heat, cold, moisture and dryness, develops this framework.

The four Khawāṣ – primary qualities of heat, cold, moisture and dryness – are used as qualitative dimensions of measurement. Heat and cold are active; moisture and dryness are passive. This concept is further developed to yield four basic universal symbols called Arkān – the primary Elements. The macrocosm – the cosmos, and its miniature – the human being, are both results of an interplay of these four Elements, which are united in unvarying patterns.

The understanding of the qualities and the Elements is an intricate and subtle idea that requires transcending gross materialism. The Elements can be perceived as components, dynamic qualities, primary forms or different phases of a cycle. However, in all these aspects the Elements represent dynamic aspects of phenomena of life, originating from one creative source.

"Life is sustained by heat and grows by moisture; heat is supported by moisture and feeds on it." Ibn Sīnā

●

(Fig. 6) Undifferentiated Reality

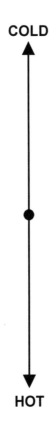

COLD

HOT

(Fig. 7) The Two Active Qualities

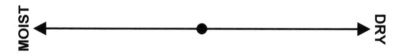

(Fig. 8) The Two Passive Qualities

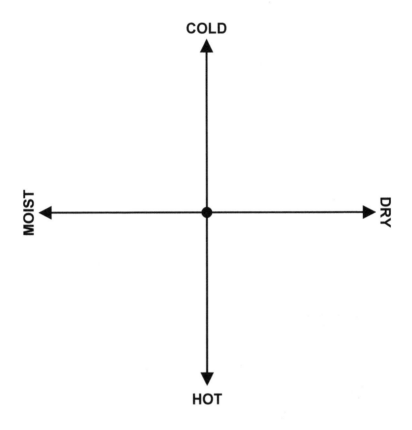

(Fig. 9) The Four Primary Qualities

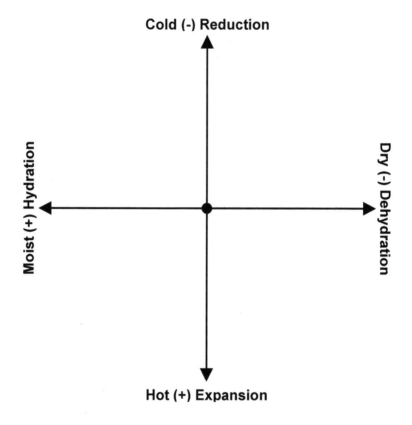

(Fig. 10) The Four Primary Qualities
and their Properties

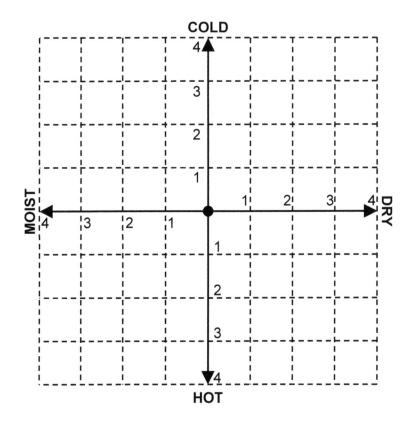

(Fig. 11) The Degrees of the Four Qualities

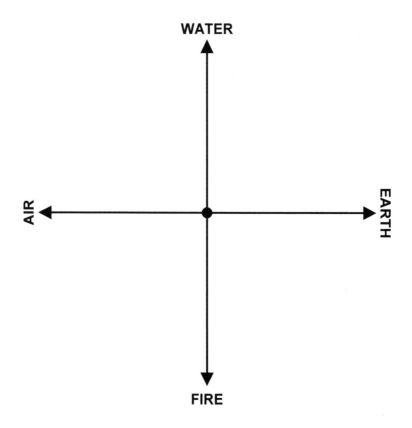

(Fig. 12) The Four Elements

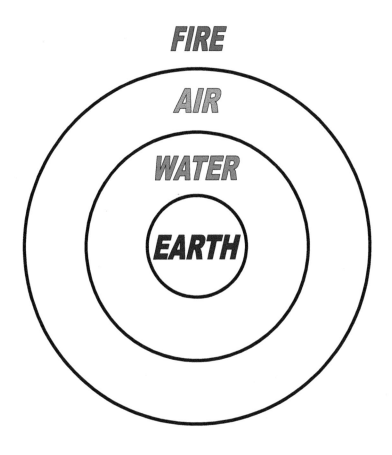

(Fig. 13) Relative Positions of the Elements

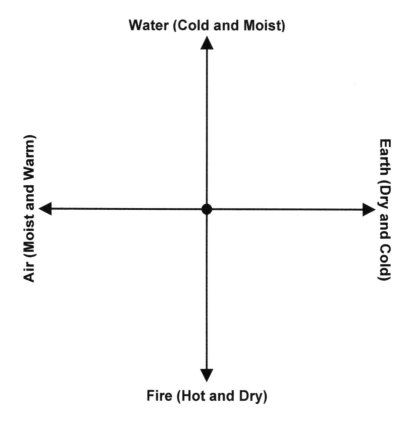

(Fig. 14) Relationship Between the

Elements and the Qualities

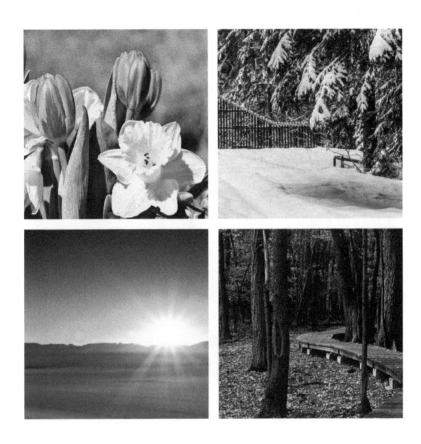

(Fig. 15) The Four Seasons Illustrated

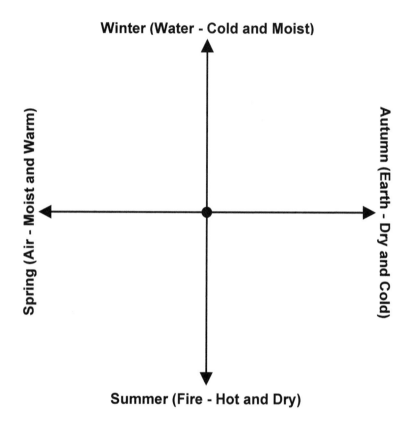

(Fig. 16) Relationship Between Seasons,
Elements and Qualities

Principles of Transformation of Qualities and Elements

Water transforms into Air by the movement of cold into heat. Air transforms into Fire by the movement of moisture into dryness. Fire transforms into Earth by the movement of heat into cold. Earth transforms into Water by the movement of dryness into moisture.

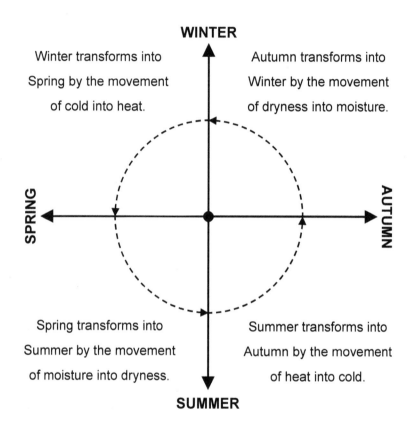

(Fig. 17) Transformation Cycle of the Seasons

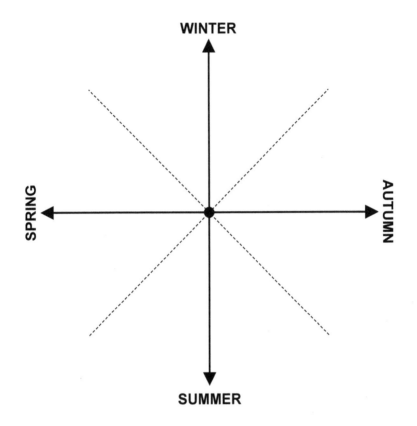

(Fig. 18) Seasons and their Divisions

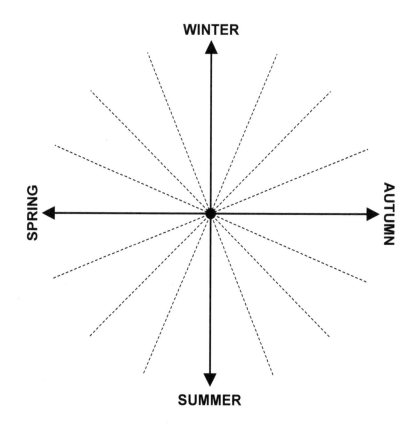

(Fig. 19) Seasons and Further Divisions

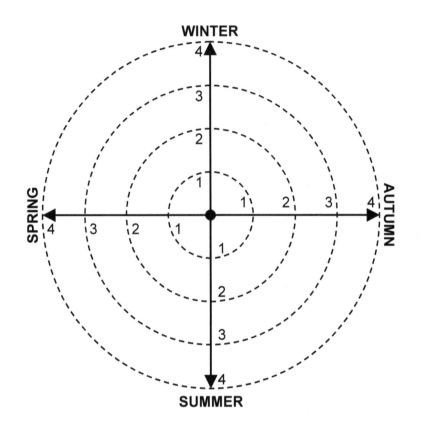

(Fig. 20) Degrees of the Seasons

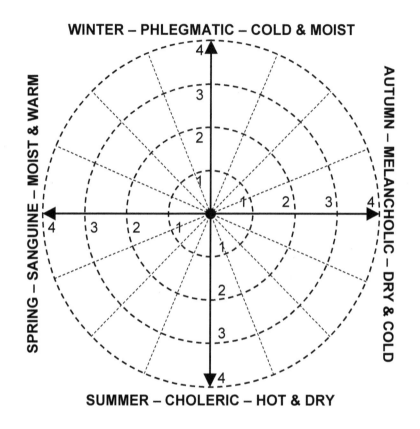

(Fig. 21) Seasons and Temperaments, their
Relationships with their Divisions and Degrees

"The Elements, Water, Air, Fire and Earth have taken their station below the heavens, each serving diligently in its own appropriate place, before or behind which it never sets foot.

Though all four are contrary in their nature and position, still one may see them ever united together. Inimical are they to each other, in essence and form, yet united into single bodies by feat of necessity. From there is born the threefold kingdom of nature." Sheikh Mahmoud Shabestari

Origin of Temperament and Hierarchy

The temperament of each individual is unique, due to inborn strengths and weaknesses of various forces. The overall temperament of the human being is hot and moist, however, variations exist depending on factors such as season, age, gender, ethnicity, occupation, emotions, habitat, and climate. Temperament is also liable to temporary changes due to these factors. [25]

(Fig. 22) Hierarchy of Temperament within the Human Being

Spectrum of Temperaments of the Whole Person

- Mu'tadil – Balanced
- Ghair Mu'tadil – Imbalanced
  - Mufrid – Singular Imbalanced [26]
    - Moist
    - Hot
    - Dry
    - Cold
  - Murākib – Complex Imbalanced [27]
    - Hot and Moist
    - Hot and Dry
    - Cold and Dry
    - Cold and Moist

Temperaments of Organs

Each part of the human body has been assigned a characteristic temperament. Thus each specific organ has hot, cold, moist or a dry temperament suitable for its structural and functional requirements. On the next page is a list of hot, cold, moist and dry organs in descending order: (1 = hottest / coldest / moistest / driest)

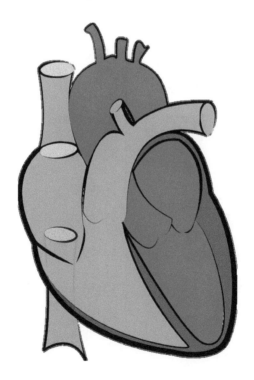

Hot	Cold	Moist	Dry
1. Vital force	1. Phlegm	1. Phlegm	1. Hair
2. Heart	2. Hair	2. Blood	2. Bone
3. Blood	3. Cartilage	3. Oil	3. Cartilage
4. Liver	4. Ligaments	4. Fat	4. Ligaments
5. Flesh	5. Tendons	5. Brain	5. Tendons
6. Muscles	6. Membranes	6. Spinal Cord	6. Membranes
7. Spleen	7. Nerves	7. Breasts	7. Arteries
8. Kidneys	8. Spinal Cord	8. Testicles	8. Veins
9. Breasts	9. Brain	9. Lungs	9. Motor Nerves
10. Testicles	10. Bones	10. Liver	10. Heart
11. Muscular coats of arteries	11. Oil of the body	11. Spleen	11. Sensory Nerves
12. Muscular coats of veins	12. Fat	12. Kidneys	
		13. Muscles	
13. Skin	13. Skin	14. Skin	12. Skin

(Fig. 23) Temperaments of Specific Organs

Dominant and Sub-Dominant Temperament

"Very few people fit perfectly into only one temperament. Most individuals have mixed temperaments. As an example, sanguine temperament as a dominant temperament and phlegmatic or bilious temperament as sub-dominant. As in nature, extremes don't exist in harmony, so it is not possible for a person who is dominant sanguine temperament to have a sub-dominant melancholic temperament." [28]

Temperament and Geographical Location

People living in the northerly countries have a moister temperament than those living in the southern countries.

Temperament and Gender

In general, females are of a colder temperament than males. [29]

Temperament and Age

Human life on Earth is divided into four periods:

1. The period of growth, which lasts up to about thirty years of age. The temperament in this period is the

most balanced in regards to heat, but moisture is in excess.

2. The prime of life, which lasts up to about forty years of age. The temperament of this age is generally hot and becoming drier.

3. The middle age, which extends to about sixty years of age. The temperament of this period is becoming colder and dry.

4. The period of decline, when weakness sets in. This lasts until death. The temperament of this period is colder and drier although on the surface it may appear moist.

The period of growth is subdivided into:

- Infancy, which is the period during which the limbs of the person are not yet fit to stand and walk.

- Babyhood, which begins when the child can stand and walk. When the deciduous teeth are giving way to permanent teeth.

- Childhood, which begins after the limbs are strong and permanent teeth have taken place. Ends at puberty.

- Juvenility (puberty), which lasts up to the appearance of hair on the face and pubes. This is when wet dreams start for males.

- Youth, which continues until growth is over. [30]

Temperament and Occupation

The temperament is more likely to be moister in people whose occupations are associated with water. The temperament is more likely to be drier in people whose occupations are associated with fire. Occupations which involve constant and excessive use of internet, computers, tablets and smartphones, are likely to develop a drier and colder temperament over time.

"The Elements are birds tied together by their feet,

Death, sickness and diseases loose their feet asunder,

The moment their feet are loose from the others

The bird of each element flies off by itself,

The repulsion of each of these principles and causes

Inflicts every moment a fresh pang on our bodies,

That it may dissolve these composite bodies of ours,

The bird of each part tries to fly away to its origin,

But the wisdom of God prevents this speedy end,

And preserved their union 'til the appointed day."

From the *Mathnāwī* by Jalāluddīn Rūmī

7. Assessment of Temperament

"It is more important to know what sort of person has a disease than to know what sort of disease a person has."
Hippocrates

The temperament of an individual is assessed against that of a balanced person under normal conditions. Since the skin, specifically the skin of the fingertips, is the most balanced, touch has been adopted as the most suitable means of assessment. However, in practice all five senses are used to arrive at a proper assessment.

There are 10 primary indicators for assessment of temperament, as follows: [31]

1. Physique
2. Complexion
3. Hair
4. Muscularity and adiposity
5. Feel of the body
6. Functional conditions of organs
7. Excretions
8. Receptivity of organs
9. Sleep and wakefulness
10. Psychological aspects

1. Physique

Individuals of hot temperament have broad chests. They have large and well developed hands and feet (not small and narrow). These people have good muscular development, especially around the joints. Their blood vessels are prominent and wide.

Persons of cold temperament have the opposite characteristics.

The characteristics of a dry temperament are dryness and roughness of the skin, and prominent joints.

2. Complexion

Paleness denotes a cold temperament. This is not to be confused with yellow complexion, as yellow indicates Yellow Bile, associated with heat.

Rosy or reddish complexion indicates excess of heat as well as abundance of blood.

A bluish tinge points to excess of cold. This is an indication that blood formation is less.

Purple colour denotes cold and dryness from the excess of Saudā – Black Bile.

Chalky colour is a sign of cold and phlegm.

Colour of the eyes can give a good indication of the temperament. Blue eyes indicate, in general, cold and moist temperament. Black eyes, in general, indicate cold and dry. Brown eyes, in general, indicate hot and dry. Grey eyes, in general, indicate hot and moist.

3. Hair

a)   Rate of Hair Growth

Slow hair growth, or lack of hair growth, is a sign of excessive cold. Rapid growth of hair is a sign of heat. When heat and dryness are present together, the hair becomes thick and profuse and grows more rapidly. Thin and scanty hair is a sign of the cold and moist temperament.

b)   Shape of Hair

Curliness indicates hot and dry temperament.

c)   Colour of Hair

Dark colour hair points to a hot temperament, and light colour hair indicates cold temperament. Grey hair points to a cold temperament, as is the case with old people.

It must be remembered that the colour of hair is also influenced by habitat and climate.

d) Excess and Scantiness of Hair

Excess of hair can be a sign of excessive Black Bile.

4. Muscularity and Adiposity

If the body is muscular, the temperament is likely to be hot and moist. In such cases, the body feels firm and solid to touch. Poor muscular development along with deficiency of fat indicates dryness. Fat and oiliness of skin point to a cold and moist temperament.

Leanness of the body is most marked in cases of excessive cold, or in cases of dryness with a balance of heat and cold, or in cases of heat with balanced dryness and moisture.

5. Feel of the Body

The temperament of a person is assessed by comparing the feel of their body with that of a normal person under normal climatic and atmospheric conditions. If feel is the same in both cases, their temperament is balanced. It may however, be relatively hot or cold.

When a person of a balanced temperament, as an assessor, finds that the feel of another individual is hot or cold, and dry or moist, this indicates that particular temperament in the person being assessed.

6. Functional Conditions of Organs

As long as the functions are performed in a natural, well integrated and whole manner, the temperament is well balanced.

Overactive and exaggerated functions, such as rapid growth and movements indicate excess of heat e.g. rapid development of organs, and rapid growth of hair.

Weakness and sluggishness of functions is a sign of cold temperament.

A hot temperament can also produce weak and sluggish movements but in that case disturbance of physical functions is generally the result of associated weakness.

Functions are reliable indication of temperament. When these are normal, and healthy, the temperament is balanced. Inferences can be made of hot, cold, dry and moist temperament from the functional state of organs.

Functions which point to heat are: a loud and powerful voice, continuous and rapid speech, short temper, brisk movements, and frequent blinking. These are signs not only of general heat in the body but also of heat in the corresponding organs.

7. Excretions

The conditions of excretions, for example, stools, urine and sweat, also indicate the energetic state of the body. Thus, strong odours, high colour full maturity and proper consistency of excretions are signs of heat. The opposite features denote cold.

8. Receptivity of Organs

Parts of the body which get quickly warmed have a hot temperament, and vice versa. This is natural because a change is acquired more easily in the direction of the existing temperament than in the opposite direction.

9. Sleep and Wakefulness

Moderation in sleep and wakefulness indicates a balanced temperament. Excessive sleep indicates a cold and moist temperament while excess of wakefulness points to heat and dryness.

10. Psychological Aspects

The following psychological traits indicate hot temperament:

- Optimism
- Fast intellect
- Pro-activity
- Strong anger
- Risk-taking
- Extraverted

The opposite of the above traits point to a cold temperament.

Quick resolution or disappearance of anger indicates a moist temperament. Lingering of anger indicates dryness.

Dreams

A person dreams of what is compatible with their temperament. A person with a hot temperament will dream of the Sun, fire, and heat. Dreams of water or ice points to a cold temperament.

Signs of a Balanced Temperament

1. Feel of the body is balanced in respect of heat, cold, dryness, moisture, softness and hardness.

2. Complexion ranges between pallor and redness.

3. Body build is neither too heavy nor too lean.

4. Blood vessels are neither superficial and prominent nor deeply submerged and hidden.

5. Hair is neither profuse nor scanty and neither too thick nor unduly thin. Its colour is tawny during childhood and dark at maturity.

6. Sleep and wakefulness are moderate.

7. Movements are free and easy.

8. Intellectual powers and memory are good.

9. Habits and behaviour are balanced between courage and timidity, anger and calmness, callousness and leniency, pride and humility.

10. Functions of all organs in the body are whole and correct.

11. Growth is rapid and deterioration of faculties slow.

12. Dreams are interesting and pleasing and portray cheerful and pleasant company with sweet voices and fragrant surroundings.

13. Good humour, popularity and geniality are fairly characteristic.

14. Meals are enjoyed and consumed in moderation and digested and assimilated normally.

15. Excretory functions are regular and normal.

Signs of Temporary Temperaments

Abnormal Heat

The signs of excessively hot Mizāj are:

1. Feeling of uncomfortable heat
2. Undue discomfort in fevers
3. Quick exhaustion of energy as activity flares up the heat
4. Excessive thirst
5. Burning and irritation in the pit of the stomach
6. Bitter taste in the mouth
7. Weak, quick and rapid pulse
8. Intolerance of hot foods
9. Comfort from cold things and
10. Distress in hot weather

Abnormal Cold

The signs of a temporarily cold Mizāj are:

1. Weak digestion

2. Less desire for drinks
3. Laxity of joints
4. Tendency for catarrhal conditions and phlegmatic fevers
5. Fondness for hot dishes and aversion to cold ones
6. Greater discomfort in winter.

Abnormal Moisture

The signs of a temporarily moist Mizāj are similar to those of a cold one but in addition there is:

1. Laxity
2. Excess of salivation and nasal secretion
3. Tendency towards diarrhoea and dyspepsia
4. Intolerance towards moist foods
5. Excess of sleep and
6. Puffiness of eye lids

Abnormal Dryness

The signs of a temporarily dry Mizāj are:

1. Dry skin
2. Insomnia
3. Wasting
4. Intolerance of dry foods but affinity for moist things
5. Discomfort in autumn

6. Ready absorption by the body of hot water and light oils.
[32]

Sketches of the Four Temperaments

Sanguine Temperament

This temperament resonates with the season of spring. "A man or a woman in whose body heat and moisture abounds, is said to be sanguine of complexion. Such are usually of middle stature, strong composed bodies, fleshy but not fat, great veins, smooth skins, hot and moist in feeling. Their body is hairy, if they be men they have soon beards, if they be women it were ridiculous to expect it. There is a redness intermingled with white in their cheeks. Their hair is usually of a blackish brown, yet sometimes flaxed. Their appetite is good, their digestion quick, their urine yellowish and thick, the excrements of their bowels reddish and firm, their pulse great and full. They dream usually of red things and merry conceits." [33]

Here's another sketch of the sanguine temperament.

"They have an oval face and head, moderate frame with more muscular tissues than fat. Joints are well formed and prominent, and hairs of head are thick and luxuriant. They are pleasantly warm to touch. They have good appetite, balanced and sound sleep, and good faculty of judgement. They have an optimistic, positive mental outlook, they are persuasive, extroverted, and have good social skills. They have a romantic nature, like to travel, play games, and engage in distractions. They are confident, poised, graceful and enthusiastic." [34]

Choleric Temperament

This temperament resonates with the season of summer. "We call that man choleric in whose body heat and dryness abounds or is predominant. Such persons are usually short of stature, and not fat, it may be because the heat and dryness of their bodies consumes radical moisture, their skin rough and hot in feeling, and their bodies very hairy. The hair of their heads is yellowish, red or flaxen for most part, and curls much, the colour of their face is tawny or sunburnt. They have some beards. They have little hazel eyes. Their concoction is very strong insomuch that they are able to digest more than their appetite. Their pulse is swift and strong, their urine yellow and thin. They are usually costive. They dream of fighting, quarrelling, fire and burning." [35]

Here's another sketch of the choleric temperament.

"They have sharp angular features, broad jaw, and a medium or lean build with flushed complexion. They have brilliant penetrating eyes, prominent veins, and light coloured hair which is often curly and thin. They have good digestion, and a sharp and quick appetite. They can have restless and disturbed sleep, often tending to wake up early or in the middle of the night. They are bold, daring, and dominant. They have brilliant intellect but they are impatient, irritable, and short tempered. Often, they turn into fearless and rebellious leaders." [36]

Melancholic Temperament

This temperament resonates with the season of autumn. "A melancholy person is one [in] whose body cold and dryness is predominate, and not such a one as is sad sometime as the vulgar dream. They are usually slender and not very tall, of swarthy, dusky colour, rough skin, cold and hard in feeling. They have very little hair on their bodies and are long without beards, and sometimes they are beardless with age. The hair of their heads is dusky brown usually, and sometimes dusky flaxen. Their appetite is far better than their concoction usually, by reason the appetite is caused of a sour vapour sent up by the spleen, which is the seat of melancholy, to the stomach. Their urine is pale, their dung of a clavish colour and broken, their pulse slow, they dream of frightful things, black, darkish, and terrible business." [37]

Here's another sketch of the melancholic temperament.

"They have a rectangular face or head, small beady eyes with sunken hollow cheeks. They are lean and thin, and have prominent bones, joints and veins. Their hair is dark, thick and straight. They have less body and facial hair. Their touch is dry, leathery and cool. Their appetite is variable or poor. They have difficulty falling asleep. They are analytical and detail oriented. Their retentive faculty of mind is well developed; they tend to be perfectionist, are practically efficient and dependable." [38]

Phlegmatic Temperament

This temperament resonates with the season of winter. "Such people in whom coldness with moisture abounds are called phlegmatick, yet are usually not very tall, but very fat. Some you shall find almost as thick as they are long, their veins and arteries are small, their bodies without hair, and they have but little beards. Their hair is usually flaxen or light brown, their face white and pale, their skin smooth, cold and moist in touching. Both appetite and digestion is very weak in them, their pulse little and low, their urine pale and thick, but the excrement of their bowels usually thin. They dream of great rains, water and drowning." [39]

Here is another sketch of the phlegmatic temperament.

"They have a round face with full cheeks, large moist eyes, and have a medium to large frame. They have more fatty tissue than muscular tissue. Their bones are well covered, and their veins are less visible. They are plump and they have delicate, soft skin. They are calm, and have sentimental and subjective thinking. They are emotional, sensitive, and tend to be religious. Their mind is foggy and slow." [40]

Thumbnail Sketches of the Four Temperaments

Sanguine

Sanguise = Blood.   Delicate, slim individuals with good circulation, emotionally cheerful.

Choleric

Chol = Bile.   Dark, brown-eyed, thin-set individuals, emotionally fiery and angry.

Phlegmatic

Phlegma = Mucus.   Blue-grey eyes, slackness of tissues, tendency towards excess fat, emotionally superficial, easygoing.

Melancholic

Melancholos = Black Bile. Soft, dark hair, green-grey-brown eyes, dry pale skin, constant nervous strain, hypochondria, gastro-intestinal atony, emotionally sad, bad tempered.

Guidelines for Assessing Temperament

In the table below, for each row, mark one option from A, B, C or D. Continue doing this for each row, then total and write down the number of ticks at the bottom of each column. After doing this, look at the next page to see which temperament each column corresponds to. The column in which you get the most ticks is most likely your dominant temperament. The column in which you get the second most amount of ticks is most likely your sub-dominant temperament. Have fun doing this, but you will need an experienced and trained facilitator if you wish to have a more accurate and nuanced assessment.

Types of Expression		A	B	C	D
1.	Complexion	Red, ruddy, flushed	White, chalky, pale	Yellow	Dusky, dark
2.	Build	Heavy, joints well developed	Flabbiness, laxity of joints	Lean / medium	Lean / thin
3.	Eyes	Red tinge	White	Yellow tinge	Dull or piercing
4.	Tongue	Red	White	Dry, yellow	Dark
5.	Mouth Tastes	Sweet	Moist	Dry	Metallic / bitter
6.	Thirst	Excessive	Lack of thirst	Excessive with dryness	Lack of thirst with dryness

7.	Appetite and Digestion	Good appetite, quick digestion	Weak appetite, weak digestion	Good appetite, strong digestion	Moderate appetite, poor digestion
9.	Sleep	Moderate	Increased	Less sleep	Poor sleep
10.	Perception	Active	Slow	Acute	Anxiety or Dullness
11.	Excretions	Prone to bleeding e.g. gums, nosebleeds	Prone to pale urine and thick saliva	Prone to diarrhoea and high colour urine	Prone to excretions with strong odours, and thin urine
12.	Dreams	Blood, red items	Water, rain, cold, snow, rivers	Fire, yellow	Dark objects, fearful places
13.	Skin	Prone to pimples and boils	Cold and moist, whitish	Dry, yellow tinge	Dry, rough
14.	Pulse	Full	Soft, slow	Rapid, thin	Weak
15.	Feel better with	Yawning and stretching	Heat, summer	Cool, moist, winter	Warmth
16.	Feel worse at	Spring (3 to 9 am)	Winter (9pm to 3am)	Summer (9am to 3pm)	Autumn (3pm to 9pm)
17.	Hair	Thick, luxuriant	Lighter colour, thin	Curly	Less hair, darker
	Score				

Answers

The column in which you get the most ticks is most likely your dominant temperament. The column in which you get the second most amount of ticks is most likely your sub-dominant temperament.

A = Sanguine (Hot and Moist)

B = Phlegmatic (Cold and Moist)

C = Choleric (Hot and Dry)

D = Melancholic (Cold and Dry)

Oneness and Diversity of Temperaments

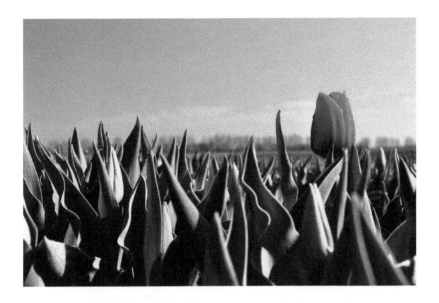

This picture illustrates the uniqueness of an individual.

(Fig. 24) One in a Million!

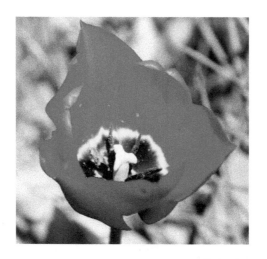

The idea of the temperament is very simple and profound. However, in practice there are many layers to each individual. This close-up picture of the red flower is one way of visualising the complexity within the simplicity. When the flower is viewed close-up, it reveals different aspects of its complexity.

(Fig. 25) Unfolding the Layers of Temperament

8. Transforming Your Health with the Four Temperaments

"He erected heaven and established the balance, so that you would not transgress the balance.   Give just weight – do not skimp in the balance." The Healing Qur'an (55:5-7)

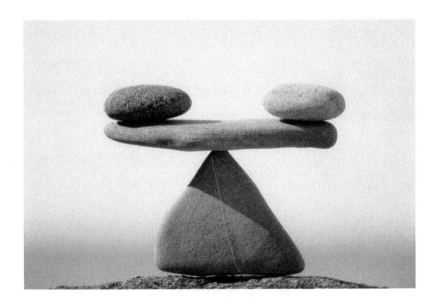

"Health is a dynamic condition of balance that is the result of an individual's ability to cope with internal and external influences. The individual needs not only to create an internal balance within him but to adapt to social, ecological and spiritual conditions." M Salim Khan

Maintaining and Restoring Balance

Having arrived at the assessment of the person's temperament, we are now in a position to understand the qualitative nature of various aspects of creation.

Every person is influenced and affected by each and every aspect of creation. This includes natural cycles and rhythms, various lifestyle factors, and human-made materials and conditions. Each of these aspects has its own energetic qualities.

In order to maintain or restore lost balance within the person, we need to utilise specific interventions to correct the imbalance.

The principles used are:

1. If the individual's temperament is in a state of equilibrium, the principle is to maintain and preserve balance. This is achieved through like or similar principle. [41]

2. If the individual's temperament is out of balance, the principle is to restore balance through application of contrary principle. [42]

The Lamp of Life

In Unani Tibb, human life and health is compared to an oil lamp made up of Innate Heat – the flame of life, and Radical Moisture – the oil that feeds the flame.

The innate heat and radical moisture of the person begins to decrease after the prime of life. There are a number of factors that can affect this process, depending on the individual's endowed temperament and lifestyle. Various physical, psychological activities, occupation and habitat also play a role in this complex process.

There is a continuous loss of radical moisture and innate heat, due to living on Earth. This is the movement, or journey, towards individual death. This movement towards natural death is destined for each person, and varies according to an individual's endowed temperament and their management of their self.

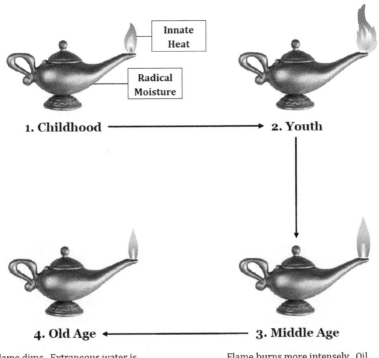

1. Childhood ⟶ **2. Youth**

Innate Heat

Radical Moisture

4. Old Age ⟵ **3. Middle Age**

Flame dims. Extraneous water is produced due to reduction in innate heat.

Flame burns more intensely. Oil maintains the flame but no longer in excess to provide for growth

(Fig. 26) The Lamp of Life

Lifestyle Balance

"If we could learn how to balance rest against effort, calmness against striving, quiet against turmoil, we could assure ourselves of joy in living and psychological health for life."
Josephine Rathbone

Preservation of both Innate Heat and Radical Moisture is necessary for maintenance of health and wellbeing. Lifestyle imbalances in their various forms cause stress to the body, mind, emotions and spirit, which accelerates the depletion of these two treasures.

In an imbalanced lifestyle, the person is 'burning the candle at both ends' and excess 'oil' is used up too rapidly. This can be manifest outwardly or the individual can 'burn on the inside'. After a period of stress, a lot of 'oil' has been used up thus the 'flame of life' dwindles. Hectic modern lifestyle accelerates ageing in this way.

See the next page for an illustration of this process using the visual metaphor of the Lamp of Life.

1. **Before Stress**

2. **During Stress**

3. **After Stress**

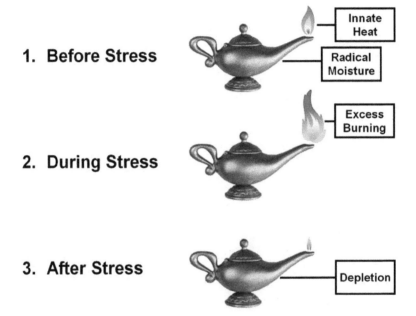

(Fig. 27) Effects of Lifestyle Imbalance
and the Lamp of Life

Heating Stimuli

- Moderate quantity of food
- Moderate amount of physical exertion
- Moderate amount of mental activity
- Moderate use of hot baths
- Moderate amount of massage
- Vigorous exercise for a short period
- Hot types of food and drink
- Hot types of medicines
- Hot types of occupations
- Dry cupping, not wet type
- Hot applications of plasters
- Moderate amount of wakefulness
- Moderate amount of sleep
- Moderate amount of pleasurable activity
- Anger
- Mild anxiety or worry, not severe
- Increased density of the skin

Cooling Stimuli

- Excessive activity, as it causes dispersion of internal innate heat

- Excessive repose, which induces cold, due to lessening of innate heat
- Excess of food and drink
- Excessive worry
- Extreme reduction of food
- Excessive joy or pleasure
- Cold types of foods and drinks
- Cold occupations
- Cold types of medicines
- External use of extreme hot items, such as water or air, due to excessive dilation of capillaries
- Prolonged applications of moderately hot things e.g. a hot bath
- Application of cooling things
- Undue increase in the density of the skin, which causes inward contraction of innate heat
- Applications of things which temporarily warm are intrinsically cold
- Undue retention of excretions which subdue innate heat
- Excessive depletions of vital fluids
- Immaturity of humours, due to lack of digestion

Moistening Stimuli

- Rest
- Sleep
- Retention
- Elimination of drying matters or activities
- Excess of foods
- Drinks of moist quality
- Foods of moist quality
- Activities which lead to increase of moisture e.g. bathing after meals
- Cold applications which increase the moisture
- Applications which moderately liquefy the body secretions
- Moderate degree of pleasure

Drying Stimuli

- Activity
- Wakefulness
- Excessive evacuations
- Inadequate food
- Foods of dry type
- Sexual intercourse
- Medicines of dry type
- Repeated emotional outbursts

- Drying applications by salt baths
- Exposure to cold
- Excessively hot applications which lead to excessive dissipation of moisture (refer to note 5 for further information).

Temperaments and Lifestyle Management

Having arrived at an assessment of one's temperament, here are some guidelines to maintain one's balance and to restore balance when lost, through appropriate management of the Asbāb-e-Sittah-Ḍharūriyya – Six Lifestyle Factors.

As a principle, for example, if an individual has a hot and dry temperament at a given time, it would not be suitable for them to be subject a lifestyle that causes heat and/or dryness. Instead, they should engage themselves in a lifestyle which promotes coolness and moisture, in order to bring them closer towards balance.

Sanguine Temperament

In order to remain healthy, they should adopt the following lifestyle factors:

Air and Environment: Avoid staying for long in hot and moist air. They can tolerate cold easily.

Food and Drink: They should preferably drink cold water and avoid excessive sugar, rich fatty foods and meat consumption. Moderation in eating habits is essential.

Physical Activity and Rest: Inadequate rest and strenuous activities should be avoided. Light weight training and aerobics for 15-20 minutes are suitable for this temperament.

Mental Activity and Rest: Excessive excitement, worry, anger or emotional excesses for kind of temperament should be avoided, deep and breathing exercise is beneficial.

Retention and Elimination: High fibre in diet in order to maintain regular bowel habits is essential, increase water intake in order to maintain regular functioning of kidney. Wet cupping twice a year (preferably in spring or summer) is recommended.

Sleep and Wakefulness: 6-7 hour of sound sleep is essential, taking sleep more than 8 hours may be harmful.

Imbalance predisposes them to diseases like uraemia, gout, diabetes, high cholesterol, reduced intestinal motility, respiratory catarrh, asthma, genito-urinary disorders, hypersensitivity, and capillary congestion. [43]

Choleric

Air and Environment: Increase in the temperature of air affects them the most, exposure to sun or hot climate should be avoided. They should live in cool, fresh and properly ventilated environment.

Food and Drink: They should avoid salt, salty foods, fats, fried foods, sour or fermented foods, excessive hot spices, chillies, excessive beef and red meat and should include milk and dairy products and cool drinks in their diet.

Physical Activity and Rest: They should avoid excessive movement and strenuous exercise, time of exercise should be early in the morning or late in the evening.

Mental Activity and Rest: Extreme emotions of anger, irritability, excessive talkativeness, and suppression of anger are emotional extremes for this kind of temperament.

Retention and Elimination: Drink plenty of water in order to eliminate heat and toxins, seasonal fruits are also beneficial.

Sleep and Wakefulness: A good night sleep for 6-8 hours is essential for such type of temperament as it is hard to get sleep, short siesta after lunch may also be beneficial.

Imbalance predisposes them to fevers, infections, rashes, urticaria, hyperacidity, headaches, migraines, eyestrain, hypertension, stress, and cardiovascular disorders. [44]

Melancholic

Air and Environment: Dry air negatively affects them. They should avoid staying in cold and dry environmental conditions for long. They need to be protected in dry weather conditions. If possible to choose their habitat, seashore and coastal areas are beneficial for their health.

Food and Drink: Melancholics should avoid old, dry and stale food, excessive beans, nuts, astringent foods, peanuts, tomatoes, eggplant (brinjal), rancid fats and nuts are harmful for them even in small quantities. Tea, coffee, artificially flavoured drinks should be avoided.

Physical Activity and Rest: Moderate and light exercise for short durations are best suited for such temperaments; especially walking first thing in the morning, as well as a short walk after dinner.

Mental Activity and Rest: Feeling of loneliness, depression and grief can have much more negative influence especially if prolonged or excessive.

Retention and Elimination: They should prevent over drying by applying moisturizers on their skin. Drink about 2 litres of water. Bodily wastes like urine and stool should never be suppressed.

Sleep and Wakefulness: They should go to bed early for 7-8 hours night sleep. They are more prone to insomnia, 10- 15 minutes break after lunch is beneficial.

Imbalance may cause anorexia, poor appetite, constipation, colon and gas related ailments, wasting, emaciation and dehydration, arthritis, neuromuscular disorders, and anxiety. [45]

Phlegmatic Temperament

Air and Environment: Cold air negatively affects them hence air conditioners and cold and wet environment should be avoided.

Food and Drink: Milk and dairy products, cheese, refined sugar and starches, glutinous foods like wheat and flour cold foods, ice-cold foods, and drinks, creamy rich foods should be avoided. But they can easily warm, hot and spicy foods.

Physical Activity and Rest: Lack of exercise and unnecessary rest during day time especially one hour before sunset should be avoided. They should indulge in strenuous exercise for longer duration. Aerobics or weight training is beneficial for them.

Mental Activity and Rest: Fear, shyness, depression are the emotional excesses for this temperament which should be managed accordingly.

Retention and Elimination: Sweating is beneficial, it should never be suppressed and warm water is also beneficial.

Sleep and Wakefulness: Sleeping for 6-7 hours is sufficient, more than this will harm them. They should get up early in the morning and avoid sleep after sunrise.

Imbalance predisposes them to phlegm congestion, water retention, oedema, slow digestion, weight gain, obesity, poor venous circulation, tendency towards depression. [46]

Temperamental Characteristics of Seasons

"Whoever wishes to pursue the science of medicine properly must proceed thus: First he ought to consider what effect each season of the year can produce, as the seasons are not alike but differ widely both in themselves and at their changes." Hippocrates

Spring is the season when leaves and flowers blossom and fruits being to be formed. Spring is of a balanced temperament. Summer is a hot and dry season. This is because excess heat evaporates moisture, and also there is generally less rain and humidity. Winter is characterised by cold and moist, opposite of summer. Autumn is cold and dry opposite of spring.

Seasonal Effects

Every season has its own specific rules provided it continues to retain its natural quality. The end of a season and the beginning of the next one are governed by the same rules and produce similar types of diseases.

Spring

Spring is normally the best season as its temperament is suited to the temperament of the vital force and blood.

Although spring is evenly balanced as mentioned above, it tends to readily change and incline towards the light cosmic heat and natural moisture. It makes the complexion rosy by drawing blood toward the surface of the skin but it does not produce dispersion as excessive heat does. During spring chronic diseases are activated by the movement and flow of dormant humours. It is for this reason that depression of melancholia becomes agitated during this season. Persons fond of excessive eating but of sedentary habits develop excessive humours during winter and in spring are predisposed to disease caused by the liquefaction and agitation of humours. When spring is prolonged there is considerable reduction in the incidence of summer diseases. Spring is called the period of the beginning and development of life.

Diseases of Spring

Bloody stools, agitation of melancholia caused by Saudā, inflammation, carbuncles, fatal forms of throat affections, boils and abscesses, rupture of vessels, and troublesome cough are characteristic maladies of this season especially when it is also cold like winter. In this type of spring, patients already are suffering from these diseases may get worse. Since the spring activates phlegmatic secretions, it produces joint pains.

The factors which aid the appearance of disease in this season are:

- Excessive physical and mental activity.
- Consumption of hot dishes.

The best way of preventing disease of this season is to carry out elimination, restrict food and ensure abundant intake of fluids.

Summer

Summer is called the period of luxurious growth. Summer disperses humours and vital forces and thus enfeebles the faculties and their functions. Blood and phlegm both decrease in this season but bile increases. Towards the end of summer, Saudā predominates because the thinner portion of bile is dispersed by heat and the heavier part is left behind as Saudā. Old persons and those resembling them look strong and healthy in summer. Summer turns the complexion yellow as the blood brought to surface is dispersed soon. During this season, diseases are generally of short duration. The reason for that is as the general vitality is good, air helps resolution by maturing and eliminating humours; but when it is low, the summer heat relaxes the tissues and produces debility. Dry summer shortens the course of disease while a moist one prolongs it. Moisture makes ordinary ulcers chronic. Conditions like diarrhoea and looseness of bowels are common. The greater incidence of disease in summer results from the migration of humours from the upper to the lower parts.

Diseases of Summer

These are various fevers, and painful affections of eyes and ears. A mild summer which is not very dry, almost like the spring, benefits fever patients. Heat and moisture favour sweating because heat liquefies the morbid humours and moisture opens up the pores by relaxation. A summer which is inclined to be cold and dry, is generally healthy but diseases caused by chill are more frequent because secretions liquefied by internal or external heat are squeezed by the prevailing cold. Diseases produced by chill are the various catarrhal conditions such as common cold and its complications. A dry type of summer benefits phlegmatic, but persons of bilious temperaments are apt to suffer from dry type of conjunctivitis and chronic type of hot fever in this type of summer. In dry summer Saudā becomes prominent from the combustion of bile, which is so readily available in this season.

Autumn

The months of autumn are called the period of tranquillity of conduct. During autumn, diseases are more frequent because of:

- Exposure to the wide fluctuations of heat and cold.
- Excessive consumption of fruit, which causes derangement of humours.
- Debility from the preceding summer carried on to this season.
- Heat producing quick and easy dispersion of the lighter portion of food, which is generally unwholesome in the season, makes the humours abnormal.
- Cold reduces dispersion and elimination of humours and diverts the humours inwards.

Blood is scanty during autumn. This is because autumn is qualitatively opposed to the temperament of blood hence it fails to replace the blood dissipated and destroyed during summer. Summer burns the humours and produces bile which autumn cools and thus produces Saudā.

Diseases of Autumn

The diseases of autumn are dry eczema, ringworm, cancer, joint pains irregular fevers. Spleen may be enlarged during autumn. The wide fluctuations of heat and cold affect the temperament of bladder. Since cold diverts the thin humours inwards and bowels tend to be loose. Sciatica also develops in this season. Bilious and irritative swellings of throat are more common in this season just as phlegmatic swellings in spring: both being due to the activation of humours from the preceding season. Occasionally coma, diseases of lungs, pain in the back and thighs also occur. The reason is that morbid humours, activated by summer, are squeezed into the tissues by the cold of oncoming winter. Mental and emotional problems are common because Saudā gets mixed with abnormal Yellow Bile humour. Ulceration of lungs is badly affected.

Autumn provides favourable opportunity to diseases, which did not appear during summer. An ideal autumn is the one, which is moist and rainy. A dry autumn is particularly harmful.

Winter

The months of winter are called the period of closing and storing. Winter aids digestion because:

- Cold aggregates the essential substance of innate heat within the body and thus makes it stronger and less prone to dispersion.
- Less fruit consumed during this season.
- Food is of more natural type.
- There is less movement and activity after meals.
- There is greater tendency to remain in warm places.

Winter is the most effective season for reducing bile because it is cold and has shorter days and longer nights. Since winter has a greater tendency to stagnate morbid matter there is a greater need of liquefying and resolving foods.

Diseases of Winter

These are generally phlegmatic in nature. Swellings, which appear during this season, are generally of a pale white colour. Cold and its complications are common in this season. When there is breeze, colds occur followed by pleurisy, pneumonia, and hoarseness of voice, pain and other affections of throat.

When winter is fully established, pain in the chest, sides, back and loins, and nervous disorders, such as chronic headache and occasionally begin to develop from excessive accumulation of phlegmatic excrements. During the season, urine is more profuse. Winter is troublesome for the old and debilitated persons, but it is beneficial for the young and healthy.

The Four Seasons in the Day and Night Cycle

The four seasons is a central theme in natural cycles. In the northern hemisphere, approximate dates for the seasons of the year are:

- Spring starts 20th March
- Summer starts 21st June
- Autumn starts 22nd September
- Winter starts 21st December

The four seasons can also be observed in a 24-hour period, in the day and night cycle. Assuming that day and night are of equal length, the seasons of the day are:

- 'Spring' in the morning from 3am to 9am
- 'Summer' in the day from 9am to 3pm
- 'Autumn' in the afternoon / evening from 3pm to 9pm
- 'Winter in the night from 9pm to 3am

The key to synchronisation with natural cycles is that the individual needs to attune themselves to these rhythms. As an illustrative example, catching the spring of the day.

Spring - like the spring season, the spring period (morning) has similar qualities. Therefore, a balanced person would be up and benefitting from the abundance of warmth and moisture during this time of the day where life is springing forth.

Summer - like the summer season, the summer period (mid-day) has the qualities of hot and dry. At this time of the day, people who have a hot and/or are living in a hot climate should be mindful of the peak heat at this time.

Autumn - like the autumn season, the autumn period (evening) has the qualities of cold and dry. This time of the day is for remaining quiet and collected.

Winter - like the winter season, the winter period (night) has the qualities of cold and moist. This time is for sleep, similar to the phenomena of hibernation in the winter season.

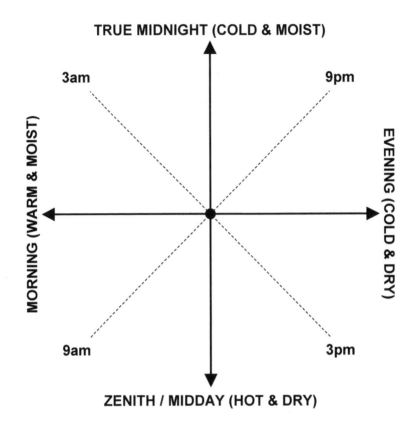

(Fig. 28) Synchronisation with Natural Cycles
in Relation to the Times of the Day and Night

Temperaments, Foods and Drinks

In Unani Tibb, each food type is classified as heating or cooling, with levels of moisture or dryness. This classification refers to the inherent temperament associated with the foods and the effect they have on the temperament of the individual.

This concept of heating and cooling food is linked to the effect of the food on the body. Foods that are heating in nature (temperament), will increase the rate of metabolism. Conversely, foods that are cooling in nature will reduce the body's metabolic rate. [47]

Tastes, Key to Understanding Foods and Drinks

Taste	Examples	Mizāj	Actions
Sweet	sugar, honey, raisins, fennel, liquorice	moderate	nutritive, ripening, softening
Bitter	dandelion, myrrh, aloe, bitter gourd, fumaria	warm and dry	cleansing, promotes heat and dryness, prevents putrefaction
Salty	salt, kelp	hot and dry	cleansing, promotes heat and moisture, prevents putrefaction
Pungent	black pepper, garlic, ginger	hot and dry	promotes heat and dryness, dissolving, lacerating

Sour	lemon, lime, hibiscus, plum	cold and dry	cooling, lessens yellow bile, digestive, promotes appetite, harmful to nerves and joints in excess
Astringent	triphola	cold and dry	promotes black bile, retentive, constipating, acts on the surface of the tongue
Acrid or Insipid	unripe fruit	cold and dry	astringent action, acts on outer and inner aspects of the tongue
Oily or Greasy	ghee, animal fats, meat, vegetable oils	warm and moist	softening and reduces appetite
Bland	water	cool and moist	reduces dryness and heat, reduces thirst, lessens yellow bile

Having arrived at an assessment of one's temperament, and having understood lifestyle guidelines for each temperament, food and drink in particular is a very important factor to health preservation and restoration.

Just as with lifestyle, the principle remains the same, that for example, if an individual has a hot and dry temperament at a given time, it would not be suitable for them to consume foods and drinks that cause heat and/or dryness, such as black coffee and garlic. Instead, they should use foods and drinks which promote coolness and moisture, such as coconut water, in order to bring them closer towards balance.

As another example, if an individual has a cold and moist temperament, it would not be suitable for them to use foods and drinks which produce coldness and moisture, such as dairy products. Instead, they should use foods and drinks which will increase their levels of warmth, such as fresh ginger tea.

Temperaments of Foods and Drinks – Examples

Category	Garam – Heating or Stimulating Foods	Sard – Cooling or Sedating Foods
Meat & Fish	Lamb, liver, rooster, goose, fish, goat (male), eggs, most birds	Goat (female), rabbit, beef
Dairy	Cheese, cream, clarified butter (ghee)	Goat's milk, cow's milk, milk, butter, yoghurt, margarine
Vegetables & Legumes	Onion, garlic, mustard, eggplant (aubergine), chickpeas, red and green peppers, turnip, parsley, radish	Lettuce, celery, Brussels sprouts, spinach, cabbage, carrot, cucumber, tomatoes, peas, potatoes, broccoli, asparagus
Fruits	Dates, figs, olives, dried fruit, raisins, ripe mangoes	Apple, melon, watermelon, mulberries, banana, peach, pear, coconut, pomegranate, apricot, plum, orange, lime, lemon

Nuts & Seeds	Sesame, almonds, pistachio, walnut, pine nuts, peanuts, hazelnut	None
Grains	Wheat, oats	Barley, maize, rice
Oils	Sunflower oil, sesame oil, mustard oil, almond oil, olive oil	Coconut oil, maize oil
Beverages	Coffee, black tea, green tea, cocoa	Coconut water, pomegranate juice
Herbs	Cinnamon, fenugreek, saffron, garam masala, most spices	Coriander, henna, rose, jasmine
Others	Honey, salt, gur, most sweet things	Refined sugar, vinegar, sour things, water

Unlocking True Health and Wellbeing

The scholars and physicians of Unani Tibb have identified and developed a comprehensive approach and framework which provides a meaningful, practical way of assessing, establishing and maintaining life balance according to a person's individual temperament.

This can be used to help design an individual's lifestyle to be in balance and harmony with rhythms and dynamics in nature that each person is subject to. This framework is known as the Asbāb-e-Sittah-Ḍharūriyya (Six Essential Lifestyle Factors). The conscious management of these six factors is fundamental to designing a wholesome lifestyle that supports positive health and wellbeing.

The Asbāb-e-Sittah-Ḍharūriyya are as follows:

- Hawā' (Air and Environment / Ecological Conditions)
- Mākūlāt-o-Mashrūbāt (Food and Drink / Diet and Nutrition)
- Ḥarakat-o-Sukūn Badanī (Physical Activity and Rest)
- Ḥarakat-o-Sukūn Nafsānī (Mental Activity and Rest)
- Istifrāgh-wa-Iḥtibās (Retention and Elimination)
- Nawm-o-Yaqẓa (Sleep and Wakefulness)

The Life Balance Wheel Activity

Begin to use the Six Essential Lifestyle Factors to assess balance or imbalance in your own life. On the next page, do the following:

1. Label each of the six sectors of the Life Balance Wheel with one each of the Six Lifestyle Factors listed on the previous page.

2. Rank the level of balance in each area in your life by drawing on the dotted line and shading in each sector. Number one being the least balanced, and ten being the most balanced.

3. Select one out of the Six Lifestyle Factors to focus on first. Write down a plan to make the necessary improvements to your lifestyle in the light of your unique temperament, taking into account the guidance and resources provided in this chapter.

4. Once you have developed life-affirming habits in one area of your lifestyle, move on to focus on another area. Make sure that you maintain your progress in the first area, too.

5. It will usually take between 30 to 90 days for you to develop a new habit or set of habits.

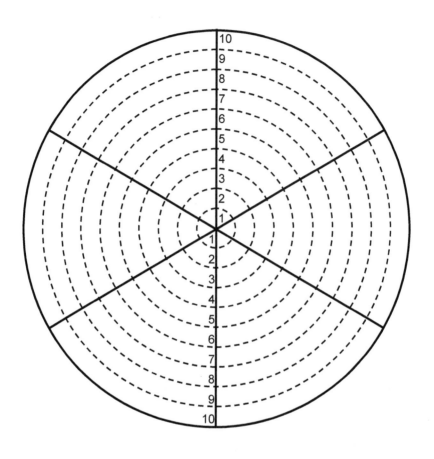

(Fig. 29) The Life Balance Wheel

"Be really whole and all things will come to you." Lao Tzu

9. Summary and Conclusions

- We live in a post-modern, post-industrial age in which the Earth is being poisoned and destroyed. Post-modern lifestyle, with all its apparent glitter and conveniences, poisons and depletes our body, mind, spirit and relationships. We are being forced away from our pure, unadulterated nature – Fiṭra, towards poor health and degenerative diseases.

- The classical civilisations of Africa, China, India, Greece and the Middle East all shared an energetic and wholistic paradigm in regards to health and well-being of human beings.

- Balance and wholeness is a central idea in all these medical traditions.

- The idea of human beings as a microcosm of the universe is also common to all of the great civilisations.

- The unity and integration of the whole person is expressed through temperaments, using the symbolic language of energy and Elements.

- The four aspects to understanding human temperament are hot, cold, dry and moist.

- Medicaments, foods, physical activities and psycho-emotional conditions all were understood in an energetic framework.
- Health and balance was maintenance of balance with all these forces and tendencies, unique to each person's own temperament.
- Today, the paradigm of synthesis and energy provides us with useful and practical ways of enhancing health and balance in ourselves and our patients.
- This framework also helps us to connect with earlier civilisations in meaningful ways and with different cultures.
- Temperament is The Golden Key that provides us with a framework for integration and ordering of knowledge in an age when there is excess emphasis on specialization and disintegration i.e. wholistic approach over the reductionist approach.
- The unitary and energetic framework helps us to restore order and balance when there is imbalance by using a range of stimuli based on energetic qualities of each intervention.

"And they will be given to drink a cup whose Mizāj (temperament) is of Zanjabīl (ginger)."

The Healing Qur'an (76:17)

Huang Ti (2697 BCE)	Yang		Yin	
Charaka Susruta (2500 BCE)	Vata	Pitta	Kapha	-
Hippocrates (460-377 BCE)	Apoplectic	-	Phlegmatic	Phthisic
Galen (138-200 CE)	Sanguine	Choleric	Phegmatic	Melancholic
Avicenna (980-1037 CE)	Hot and Moist	Hot and Dry	Cold and Moist	Cold and Dry
Halle Huson (1821 CE)	Temperamens Partiels	Cephalique	Abdominale	Thoracique
Rostan (1828 CE)	Type Musculair	Cerebral	Digestif	-
Carus (1853 CE)	Athletic	Cerebral	Phlegmatic	Asthenic
Laycock (1862 CE)	Sanguineous	Billous	Phlegmatic	Indancholic
Eppinger (1917 CE) & Hess (1931 CE)	-	Sympathetic Otonic	Vagotonic	-
Danielopolu (1920 CE)	Amphotonic	Sympathetic Otonic	Vagotonic	Amphophypo Tonic
Jung (1923 CE)	Extrovert	-	-	Introvert
Kretschmer (1926 CE)	Athletic	Dysplastic	Pyknic	Asthenic
Hurst (1927 CE)	Hyperasthenic gastric diathesis	Hypoasthenic gastric diathesis	Gall bladder diathesis	Asthma and migraine diathesis
Pavlov (1849-1935 CE)	Lively	Impetuous	Calm	Weak
Pearson and Wyllie (1935 CE)	-	Neuro arthritic	Lymphatic	-
Sheldon (1940 CE)	Ectomorph	Mesomorph	Endomorph	-

Sheldon (1940 CE)	Cerebrotonia	Somatotonia	Viscerotonia	-
Peterson (1946 CE)	-	-	Pyknic	Leptosomic
Vannier (1952 CE)	Carbonic	Phosphotic	-	Flouric
Brooks and Mueller (1966 CE)	Uric acid	-	Cholesterol	-

(Fig. 30) Historical Summary of Temperaments

"We will show them Our signs in the horizons and within themselves until it becomes clear to them that it is the truth. But is it not sufficient concerning your Lord that He is, over all things, a Witness?" The Healing Qur'an (41:53)

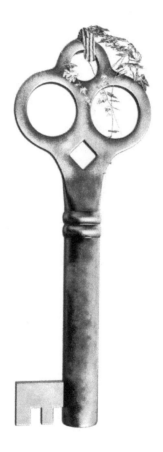

Your Journey to Higher Health

Good health is essential for a full and happy life. Perfect health means complete enjoyment of all our inherent vitality and clarity of mind; it is a state of total wellbeing and happiness. Benefit now by taking advantage of the following opportunities to improve your own health and to help others:

- **'The 7 Steps' Free Mini-Course**
  www.CoMHA.org.uk/7s

- **Life Balance & Healthy Living Programme**
  www.CoMHA.org.uk/Online

- **In-Person Programmes and Retreats**
  http://www.CoMHA.org.uk/Foundation

- **Professional Diploma in Herbal & Naturopathic Medicine (Unani Tibb)**
  E-mail admissions@CoMHA.org.uk

- **Accredited Trainer Programme**
  E-mail admissions@CoMHA.org.uk

- **Connect to Us**
  www.CoMHA.org.uk/newsletter
  www.Facebook.com/CoMHAuk
  www.LinkedIn.com/in/mohsinhealth

Glossary

Akhlāṭ

Plural of Khilṭ; the four primary humours: blood, phlegm, bile and black bile.

Arkān

Literally meaning 'pillars'. In this context, refers to the classical elements. In Unani Tibb, there are four elements: earth; water; air; and fire. This is not to be confused with the modern study of specific elements in chemistry.

Asbāb-e-Sittah-Ḍharūriyya

Literally 'the six essential causative factors' (also known as the Six Lifestyle Factors) or the theory of causes – which identifies and explains the reasons for deviations from the norms so that they may be corrected.

Balgham

Phlegm: one of the four humours, cold and moist.

Constitution

Sum of all inherited characteristics.

Dam

Blood: one of four humours, hot and moist.

Diathesis

(Greek, diathesis: condition, state.) Represents a pathological condition, disease manifestations at specific body sites.

Disposition

Susceptibility to disease.

Fiṭrah

Nature. Pure, unadulterated forms and functions such as the innocence of a new born infant.

Ḥifẓ-e-Ṣiḥḥah

Preservation or maintenance of health. (See also Ṣiḥḥah)

Ḥijāmah

Use of different types of cupping, such as dry or wet cupping, for preservation of health and treatment of diseases.

Kapha

A core Ayurvedic term which may be translated as the principle that controls structure. One of the three Doshas.

Khawāṣ

Primary qualities i.e. heat, cold, moisture, dryness.

Macrocosm

The greater cosmos.

Maraḍ

Disease, an abnormal state that primarily disturbs normal functions.

Microcosm

Human being, miniature cosmos.

Mizāj

A central idea in Unani Tibb which literally means a mixture which has an ability to remain stable for some time. In a clinical context, it is the synthesis or wholeness which expresses the individuality of a particular person.

Muʿtadil

Balance or equilibrium.

Pitta

That which controls metabolism. One of the three Doshas.

Prakruti

An Ayurvedic concept which means nature or constitution.

Quwā

Faculties, powers, energies or forces.

Ṣafrā

Yellow bile: one of the four humours, hot and dry.

Saudā

Black bile: one of the four humours, cold and dry.

Ṣiḥḥah

Health, a dynamic condition of I'tidāl – balance in which all the Af'āl – functions are carried out in a Ṣaḥiḥa – correct and Salīma – whole manner.

Ṭabī'at

Vis medicatrix naturae – The Healing Power of Nature.

Tridosha

A core Ayurvedic concept which means biological fluids of Vata, Pitta and Kapha.

Unani Tibb

Whole-person healthcare and medicine, the body of knowledge and practices that deals with the state of Insān – human beings – in health and disease. Its primary purpose is to maintain health and wellbeing, and endeavour to restore it when lost.

Vata

An Ayurvedic principle which controls movement. One of the three Doshas.

Waḥdāt

The whole of life and the human being as an integrated totality.

Yang

Literally means the sunny side of a mountain.

Yin

Literally means the shady side of a mountain.

Yin-Yang

A fundamental Chinese concept.

Notes and References

1. Current Health Crisis

[1] The Science Museum, *Thalidomide*, accessed 13th June 2018,(http://broughttolife.sciencemuseum.org.uk/broughttolife/themes/controversies/thalidomide)

[2] BBC News, 8th February 2018, *10 charts that show why the NHS is in trouble*, accessed 13th June 2018, (https://www.bbc.co.uk/news/health-38887694)

[3] Ibid.

[4] Ibid.

[5] BBC News, 3th February 2018, *'Undervalued' GPs fuelling a 'crisis'*, accessed 13th June 2018, (https://www.bbc.co.uk/news/uk-england-42905115)

2. Traditional Chinese Understanding of Temperament

[6] Huang Ti, *Huang Ti Nei Ching Suwen - The Yellow Emperor's Classic of Internal Medicine*, University of California Press, Berkeley, Los Angeles, 1972, p. 16

[7] Maciocia, G., *The Foundations of Chinese Medicine*, Churchill Livingstone, London, 1989, p. 8.

[8] Ibid.

3. Ayurvedic Understanding of Temperament

[9] Charaka, *Charaka Samhita*, Chawkham Bha Orientalia, Varnasi, 2011, p. xii

[10] Udupa, K. N, *Science and Philosophy of Indian Medicine*, Shree Baidyanath Ayurveda Bhan, Nagpur, India, 1978, p. 86

[11] "The Indian system of medicine clearly recognises the distinctions in human temperament and individual differences in psychological and moral disposition, his reaction to socio-cultural and physical environment." Ibid., p. 44

4. European Understanding of Temperament

[12] Herget, H.F., *Constitutional Medicine*, Pascoe, Giessen, 1998, p. 16

[13] Abu Asab, M., Amri, H., Micozzi, M.S., *Avicenna's Medicine*, Healing Arts Press, Rochester, Vermont, USA, 2013, p. 12

[14] Herget, op. cit., p. 13

[15] The Graeco-Arabic educational material was conveyed to central Europe via translation Colleges. Constantine the African (1015 CE - 1087 CE) translated from Arabic into Latin the text books of Ali Abbas and others. The most important translation school was Toledo, Spain. In the 12th Century the works of Avicenna and others were translated into Latin as Corpus Toletanum. The first time medical schools in the West, Salerno and Montpellier, were set up in places where Arabic culture and cultures of European middle ages met. From then on, medicine moved from private and ecclesiastical medical schools, to then universities. Ibid., p. 23

[16] Temperament from Latin Temperare, to temper, restrain, compound, moderate.

[17] Rolfe, R., *The Four Temperaments*, Marlowes Company, New York, 2002, p. 18

[18] Herget, op. cit., pp. 31-32

[19] Constitution from constitutio conporis (L.) = physical make-up as the sum of all the inherited characteristics; this medical term originates from the works of Galen. For this concept, Hippocrates tends to use the word physis (Gr.):

natural composition, structure in conjunction with katastasis and schema (condition, state). Herget, op. cit., p. 18

[20] Ibid.

5. Unani Tibb: Whole-Person Healthcare & Medicine

[21] Khan, M.S., Article: *Unani Tibb: Whole-Person Healthcare & Medicine*, Mohsin Health, Leicester, UK, 2009.

6. Unani Tibb Understanding of Mizāj – Temperament

[22] Ibn Sina, *The Canon of Medicine of Avicenna*, translated by O.C. Gruner, Augustus M. Kelley, New York, 1970, p. 34.

[23] Mizaj is derived from the Arabic word Imtizaj meaning to make a mixture. Kitab-fil-al-Mizaj, Ibn Sina Academy, Aligarh, 2008, p. 104

[24] Ibn Sina, op. cit.

[25] Humankind enjoys the most flexible temperament. Humans are surviving equally, from arctic to equatorial zones. Because of this greater range of flexibility, humankind's temperament is considered to be the most equable and appropriate, and thus termed as Mizaj-e-Ashraf – the best of all temperament. Zaid, I.H., Temperamentology, Amil, Aligarh, 1999, p. 15

[26] Simple imbalance of temperament = Su-e-Mizaj-Sada

[27] Complex and structural change in temperament = Su-e-Mizaj-Maddi

[28] Bhika, R., Prof., *Theoretical Principles of Tibb*, Ibn Sina Institute of Tibb, Roodenport, 2018, p. 37

[29] Metabolic rate varies with gender, it is lower in females. Males have BMR 40 calories, hour/square metre of body structure, whereas in females its value is 37 calories. Zaid, I.H., Temperamentology, Amil, Aligarh, 1999, p. 15

[30] Metabolic rate (MR) varies in accordance with age and is inversely proportional to the age. In younger people, base metabolic rate (BMR) as well as body fluid contents are relatively higher, thus their temperament is Har-Ratab - warm and moist. Ibid.

7. Assessment of Temperament

[31] Ibn Sina, *Al-Qanun Fil Tibb*, Jamia Hamdard, Delhi, 1993, p. 14

[32] Ibid.

[33] Tobyn, G, *Culpeper's Medicine*, Singing Dragon, London, 2013, pp. 83-88

[34] Jabin, F. A., *Guiding Tool in Unani Tibb for Maintenance and Preservation of health: A review study*, Afr. J. Tradit. Complement. Altern. Med. (2001) 8 (5): pp. 140 - 143

[35] Tobyn, G., op. cit., pp. 83-88

[36] Jabin, F. A., op. cit.

[37] Tobyn, G., op. cit.

[38] Jabin, F. A., op. cit.

[39] Tobyn, G., op. cit.

[40] Jabin, F. A., op. cit.

8. Transforming Your Health with the Four Temperaments

[41] In Tibb, health is maintained through the use of like principle. For example, for an individual who is already balanced in regards to hot and cold, they are kept in balance by providing balanced stimuli, appropriate to the individual person.

[42] Any imbalance is remedied by providing opposite stimuli. For example, excess heat is brought back to balance by providing cold stimuli of the correct degree, extent, and duration that is appropriate to the individual person.

[43] Jabin, F. A., op. cit.

[44] Ibid.

[45] Ibid.

[46] Ibid.

[47] Bikha, R. and Valles, N., *Cooking for Your Body Type*, The Ibn Sina Institute of Tibb, Roodenport, 2003, p. 9

Index

A

Africa, 1, 184

Akhlāṭ. *See* humours

Arabia, 1

Arkān. *See* Elements

Asbāb-e-Sittah-Ḍharūriyya. *See* Six Lifestyle Factors

Aschner

    haematogenic constitution, 57

    lymphatic constitution, 57

    mixed constitution, 57

autumn (fall), 110, 114, 139, 143, 144, 148

Ayurveda, 21, 41-48, 62

    Doshas, 41

    Elements, 41

    Prakruti, 41

    temperament – Kapha, 47

    temperament – Pitta, 45

    temperament – Vata, 43

    Tridosha. *See* Doshas

B

balance

    foods and drinks, 152

    Josephine Rathbone, 128

    maintaining, 125, 133

    restoring, 125, 133

C

China, 1, 62, 64, 71, 158

Chinese medicine, 21, 27-40, 28, 33, 35, 38, 62

    Five Element Theory, 35

    Nei Ching, 40

    Yellow Emperor's Classic of Internal Medicine, 29

    Yin-Yang. *See* Yin-Yang

choleric (bilious) temperament

    Element, 52

    humour, 52

    lifestyle guidelines, 134

    qualities, 52

    sketch, 113

    thumbnail sketch, 117

complementary and alternative medicine (CAM), 22

cosmology, 51

cosmos, 22, 51, 60, 62, 65, 71

D

Darwin, 54

Page 178

dehumanisation, 14, 24

Di Giovanni, 55

diet. *See* food and drink

diseases

anorexia, 137

anxiety, 137

apoplexy, 50

arthritis, 137

asthma, 134

cancers, 9, 10

capillary congestion, 134

cardiovascular, 9, 136

catarrh, 134

chronic. *See* NCDs

circulation, 138

constipation, 137

definition, 68

degenerative. *See* NCDs

dehydration, 137

depression, 138

diabetes, 9, 10, 11, 134

digestive, 138

emaciation, 137

energy depletion, 3

eyestrain, 136

fever, 136

genito-urinary, 134

gout, 134

headache, 136

heart disease, 10

high cholesterol, 134

hyperacidity, 136

hypersensitivity, 134

hypertension, 136

iatrogenic, 14

infection, 136

infections, 15

intestinal, 134, 137

lifestyle. *See* NCDs

lung cancer, 11

migraine, 136

NCDs, 3, 4, 9, 14, 58, 140,
158

neuromuscular, 137

non-communicable. *See*
NCDs

obesity, 138

oedema, 138

of autumn (fall), 143

of spring, 140

of summer, 142

of winter, 145

rash, 136

respiratory, 9

stress, 136

stroke, 10

tuberculosis, 50

tumours, 58

uraemia, 134

urticaria, 136

Page 179

water retention, 138

Western. *See* NCDs

doctors

workload pressure, 19, 20

drugs

method, 22

pharmaceutical, 4, 12

thalidomide, 12

E

economical, 62

Egyptian medicine, 49, 62

Elements (Arkān), 70, 71, 72, 80, 81, 82, 84, 85, 91, 158

Jalāluddīn Rūmī, 100

environment, 6, 10

Europe, 1, 14, 22, 23, 173

renaissance, 1, 13

European medicine, 49-58

F

Fiṭra, 3, 158

food and drink

choleric temperament, 135

cooling, 131

degradation, 10

deviation, 10

drying, 132

heating, 130

intolerance of hot foods, 109

intolerance of moist foods, 110

liquefying, 145

melancholic temperament, 136

moistening, 132

phlegmatic temperament, 137

restricting, 141

sanguine temperament, 134

tastes, 150

temperaments of, 150, 152

Fritjof Capra, 3, 21, 25, 65

G

Galen, 161, 174

germs, 13

Golden Key, 1, 69, 159

Greece, 64, 71, 158

Greek medicine, 49

H

health

balance, 124

crisis, 3, 4, 14

definition, 68

individuality, 1

design, 154

imbalance, 128, 129

management, 133

M

magic bullet, 12, 13

Maimonides, 64

materialism, 13

medical establishment, 22

medicine

definition, 68

melancholic temperament

Element, 52

humour, 52

lifestyle guidelines, 136

qualities, 52

sketch, 114

thumbnail sketch, 117

microcosm, 51, 60, 158

Middle East, 62, 64, 71, 158

Mizāj. *See* temperament

modern. *See* industrial

N

National Health Service. *See* NHS

natural cycles and rhythms, 125, 147, 149

NHS, 171

A&E targets, 18

crisis, 15

doctors, 19, 20

spend, 16, 17

nutrition. *See* food and drink

O

osteopathy, 22

P

pharmaceutical complex, 22

phlegm congestion, 138

phlegmatic temperament

Element, 52

humour, 52

lifestyle guidelines, 137

qualities, 52

sketch, 115

thumbnail sketch, 117

poverty, 4

primary qualities (Khawāṣ), 70, 71, 72, 75, 76, 77, 78, 79, 82, 84, 85

public healthcare, 4, 15, *See also* NHS

CPSIA information can be obtained
at www.ICGtesting.com
Printed in the USA
BVHW060146060319
541746BV00001B/1/P

9 780992 945619